BRAIN AND PERSONALITY

Brain and Personality

GRAHAM POWELL

PRAEGER PUBLISHERS
Praeger Special Studies

New York • London • Sydney • Toronto

PRAEGER PUBLISHERS, PRAEGER SPECIAL STUDIES
383 Madison Avenue, New York, N.Y. 10017, U.S.A.

Published in the United States of America in 1979
by Praeger Publishers
A Division of Holt, Rinehart and Winston/CBS, Inc.

Library of Congress Catalog Card Number: 79-87638

Printed in Great Britain

Contents

Foreword

A necessary prerequisite for someone to possess in order to attempt a formulation of the neuropsychology of human personality is the ability to select, organise and integrate relevant findings from the sciences of neurology and psychology both in their experimental and applied forms. Dr. Graham Powell possesses that rare combination of academic scholarship and clinical experience which permits him to embark upon this ambitious venture. The results of his endeavours are impressive, and his insights and suggestions are reasonable and stimulating . . . . beyond the data yet never the pale.

Dr. Powell evaluates, in particular, Eysenckian research and theory concerning the higher functioning of the human central nervous system and relates this to studies on the influence of varieties of brain lesions upon behaviour. The work of Luria and of Pribram upon the regulation and planning of behaviour contributes a further dimension to Dr. Powell's model. It is indeed refreshing to find a statement upon brain and personality where the neuropsychological variables are measurable and the theory testable.

It is work such as Dr. Powell's that promotes the clinical neuropsychologists' claim of being more concerned with the restoration of brain function than with the assessment of brain dysfunction i.e. the role of clinical neuropsychologist as therapist.

In 1949 Ryle's 'The Concept of Mind' and Hebb's 'Organization of Behavior' created the climate for advancement in the exploration of the 'mind/brain' problem. Thirty years on, Powell's 'Brain and Personality' should prove as seminal a publication for it is as relevant to the philosopher as it is important to the clinician . . . very!

Anthony W.H. Buffery
Senior Lecturer in Psychology,
Institute of Psychiatry,
University of London
14. 2.79.

1 An introduction and some problems

Introduction

In an article entitled 'Towards a neuropsychological theory of person', Pribram (1968) concludes by stressing the point that the individual can only be fully described by an examination and synthesis that cuts across many disciplines, otherwise the study of the person 'is likely to culminate in a tower of Babel where the many, by referring to the same event structured in different realms of discourse, fail totally to communicate'. It is the same theme which runs through much of Eysenck's work, as in his book *The Biological Basis of Personality* (1967), where in the same vein he says 'we might hope to end up with a unified psychology presenting a single face to the world rather than the present, somewhat schizophrenic, Janus-like apparition'. Also in the same vein, the purpose of this book is to describe, criticise and evaluate certain areas of brain research and certain areas of personality research that appear to overlap and have implications for each other.

The area of brain-personality relationships seems to be a much neglected field. For example, in the writings of one of the most influential figures in neuropsychology, A.R. Luria, the word 'personality' does not even merit a place in the subject index (see Luria, 1966). It has been pushed into the background by the extensive investigation of other aspects of cognitive functioning particularly memory, language, and intellectual functioning. One can only guess at why this should be. It cannot be that the brain-personality relationship is an unimportant one, since subtle personality changes are a very common occurrence after brain injury even in the absence of specific cognitive impairment. Patients tend to use phrases like 'I just don't feel myself any more', or 'I haven't got going again since the accident' or 'My wife sees the difference in me', and, as will be seen, a very high proportion of patients suffering brain assaults suffer psychiatric breakdowns. What is more, the area of brain-personality relationships should never have been allowed to become a neglected field: not when tens of thousands of psychosurgical operations have been performed and will be performed. Perhaps the reasons for neglect are sheer practical ones. It is easier to evaluate the statement 'I can't remember much any more' than to evaluate 'I don't feel myself any more', and one can see for oneself, even in a short follow-up interview, that a patient cannot talk properly or understand properly, but one cannot 'see' a subtle personality problem in the same way.

Hécaen (1964) has found that at least 21 per cent of cerebral tumour cases suffer some kind of personality change altering mood or character. As an upper limit, Lishman (1968) has found that some 87 per cent of penetration injuries cause a degree of personality breakdown. In the light of such figures, no one can deny the importance of investigation into brain-personality relationships.

An outline and some problems

The brain is a conglomeration of specialised tissue whose job it is to assist the organism in its quest for self-survival and self-reproduction. It achieves this end by forming an organised image of the environment through information collected by receptor cells, and by forming an organised response using effector units. A leaf does as much when it detects the sun and turns towards the warmth. The big difference between us and a leaf, however, is in the complexity of the stimuli we are able to detect and the complexity of responses that we are capable of emitting. It follows that there must be a greater complexity of organised processing between input and output.

With complexity, there must also come variety - more and more possible ways of organising input, mediation and output - and it is this variety that allows a consideration of individual differences between organisms, in a manner which does not, presumably, apply as much to our lowly leaf.

Individual differences in how effector response patterns (behaviours) are organised, have long been the province of personality theorists. It seems that certain specific behaviours are linked together to form superordinate dimensions, and that individuals can be placed at various points along each dimension or trait. The position of any person on a trait somehow reflects the strategy he or she uses to cope, live and ultimately survive. In other words, personality traits reflect the way that individuals are organised.

The basic premise to be considered here is now evident. It is this: if the role of the brain is to organise, and if personality traits are organisations (or a product of organisation) then it is inconceivable that personality is not ultimately a function of brain. Translating the premise into an explicit question, we have: what aspects of brain have implications for personality? This is the one question which will be asked throughout. Various properties or dimensions of brain will be taken and hopefully mapped on to properties or dimensions of personality. Broadly speaking there are four general ways of measuring brain:

1 Tissue or neuronal characteristics that might be governed by the chemical properties and activities of the cells (e.g. their general level of excitation, the ease with which they can be fired, or the number of firings they can make in a given period).

2 The intactness or efficiency of groups of cells that underlie a particular psychological function (e.g. to include the effects of brain lesions in different areas, or the level of activity within certain systems such as the limbic system or ascending reticular system).

3 The manner in which groups of cells that underlie a particular psychological function are physically distributed within and between the two cerebral

hemispheres (e.g. whether language functions are in the left or right hemisphere, or the degree of specialisation or lateralisation between the two hemispheres, or the degree of nuclear 'grouping' within a hemisphere).

4 Features of brain processing that can be considered with no reference to an organic or physical substrate (e.g. ability to form plans of action, or the degree of redundancy preferred in processing, or level of risk-taking in decision-making, or complexity of 'neural' network).

There is just one point more to make about these admittedly crude divisions. Several of the brain parameters to be considered claim to refer to one of the first three types (all three of which have some concrete link with the physical brain), whereas they would be better placed in the last category (where the items come perilously close to being as 'distant' from the organic reality of the brain as any other psychological hypothetical construct). In essence, parameters placed in the fourth category require an analysis tracing them back to the physical brain, in much the same way as is in progress here regarding personality. This issue will be picked up as we go along, in the section on Strength of the nervous system, for example.

The format of subsequent chapters will be to take a dimension or feature of brain, describe it, trace the theoretic links with personality, and then examine the empirical evidence. There are at least two major difficulties. The first is that theoretical links between brain parameters and personality are extremely hard to delineate because of the sheer distance between the two concepts; they are almost at the two extremes in terms of levels of analysis. How do you relate the way a person's neurons behave to whether or not he goes to parties? As Eysenck (1972) points out, one needs an awful lot of 'transducers' to link up phenomena in the central nervous system (CNS) with social behaviours, and there are many possible chains of argument. Some researchers, particularly the Russian school, avoid the problem altogether by studying types of nervous systems *per se*, without making any reference to real-life indices of type or any behavioural measures of personality. The Russian failure to relate explicity brain type and personality type has been succinctly criticised by Eysenck (1972), who pointed out that 'a single questionnaire measure of extraversion and neuroticism, or of Cattell's exvia and anxiety concepts, would have provided the bridge between their work and that carried out in the Western World'.

The second general difficulty concerns the preferred experimental methodology of researchers and the problem this causes when it comes to piecing together available evidence. The preference is to undertake research only on adjacent levels of analysis. There are, of course, good reasons for doing this: vocabulary and concepts are more likely to overlap, theoretical relationships are more easily perceived, there is more likely to be a body of previous work, and if relationships are found then they are more easily explainable. The problem this raises can be seen by supposing that there are three levels of analysis. A, B and C each with at least one important parameter to be assessed, *a, b* and *c* respec-

Fig. 1.1 Levels of analysis in personality research (from Eysenck 1972)

I	II	III	IV	V
Inherited differences in anatomical and physiological structures:	Psychophysiological differences:	Observed differences: Experimental studies:	Personality:	Special phenomena:
	EEG	Conditioning	Extraversion-introversion	Neurosis
Visceral brain	EMG	Learning		Crime
Reticular formation →	GSR →	Sensory thresholds →	Neuroticism-stability →	Accident-proneness
Neocortex	Uric acid			Sexual behaviour
		Perception		
	Catecholamines			
		Motivation		

tively. If one wishes to know the relationship between *a* and *c* one is liable to be faced with two studies indicating, perhaps, a positive relationship between *a* and *b*, and between *b* and *c*. This is an old problem, of course. One cannot assume that *a* and *c* are also positively related. There may be no common variance between *a* and *c* and they may account for totally different aspects of the variance in *b*. A similar problem can be stated by considering three sets of objects, *p*, *q* and *r*. If all *p*s are *q*s and all *r*s and *q*s, one still knows nothing about whether any *p*s are *r*s. The following logic is obviously erroneous:

Tortoises eat lettuce
My wife eats lettuce
∴ My wife is a tortoise

but the following logic, equally erroneous, has a deceptive appeal to which Petrie (1952) and Willett (1960) seem to have succumbed:

Extraverts have high Porteus maze error scores
Frontal lobectomies increase Porteus maze error scores
∴ Frontal lobectomies increase extraversion

The point being made is that if one wishes to relate two parameters at distant levels of analysis then there is no substitute for a study in which the two parameters are simultaneously measured. Such studies are, however, rare in the field of brain and personality. Instead we often have to fiddle around with results pertaining to shorter causal chains that have to be spliced together to give what we hope is a reasonable representation of the relationship between the two distant parameters that we are really interested in. At best, this type of evidence can only be considered 'circumstantial' and tentative. At least, it should make us aware of the distance between our evidence and our conclusion. For example, if we know that (a) caffeine improves vigilance, (b) introverts are better at vigilance tasks, then might we not conclude, really, that introverts drink more coffee? This conclusion is nearer the evidence than is one concerning the function of the ascending reticular activating system, which might otherwise be offered.

One of the most common ways used to get around the inadequacy of such evidence is to pile up the number of similarities that are detectable between two concepts or dimensions, and present them in a nice table. See, for example, how Gray (1964) tries to establish links between arousal, and strength of the nervous system, or between equilibrium in dynamism, and extraversion (1967). To return to my wife and the tortoise, one could point out that behaviourally they are both most active before eating, both appreciate a long snooze in the morning, and both enjoy a good long walk; emotionally they are both affectionate and good-tempered (neither bite when provoked). However long this list is extended, I still cannot believe that I am married to a tortoise. In sum, one or two crucial differences can outweight any number of similarities. This emphasis on the search for disconforming evidence is otherwise known as divergent validity in the sphere of assessment theory (Wiggins, 1973). For instance, in relation to the previous example concerning extraverts, mazes and lobectomies, it matters not a whit that extraverts and lobectomised patients both draw lines inaccurately, both have low self-blame scores, both have low physical endurance, both have an increased interest in the present (Petrie, 1952), if the lobectomised individuals do not exhibit the behavioural features that are the core of extraversion, such as being chatty, having many friends and liking going to parties.

These problems will be returned to as specific examples arise. They reflect, of course, nothing more than a lack of extensive information about brain and personality relationships, but this is not to suggest a certain futility in the present literary endeavour before it really starts. Rather, although it must be accepted that we only have a glimmering of understanding, these glimpses of relationships are exciting. They expand our knowledge of both brain and personality. Above all they push psychology towards examining the organism as a whole, at all levels.

2 Cortical excitation and inhibition: Eysenck's theory

The first aspect of brain to be considered here concerns two fundamental states of neurons, of neuronal networks, and of the cortex as a whole. They are (a) the excitatory state, in which individual neurons, networks, or the whole cortex are activated or in a condition that is primed and ready for action, (b) the inhibitory state, where neurons, neural networks, or all the cortex are inert and less easily activated.

Eysenck's (1957) neurophysiological and neuropsychological theory relates individual differences in the patterning and modulation of these two states to the extraversion-introversion dimension of personality. The extravert is sociable, outgoing and gregarious; liking change and preferring action to thought — and is paradoxically predicted to be in an inhibited state cortically. Introverts keep their own company, either because they prefer it or because they are a little afraid of others; they do not need a constant changing of activities and are reflective rather than impulsive — but are paradoxically predicted to be in a cortically excited state.

As will be seen, the interplay between excitation and inhibition is largely regulated by the brain-stem mechanism known as the reticular activating system (RAS): the oldest and most basic part of our central brain.

Statement of theory

In the *Dynamics of Anxiety and Hysteria*, Eysenck (1957) lays down two postulates to account for the introvert-extravert dimension of personality. The first postulate clearly places the theory within the realm of physical neural processing, and hence within the scope of this book. It is:

> Human beings differ with respect to the speed with which excitation and inhibition are produced, the strength of the excitation and inhibition produced, and the speed with which inhibition is dissipated. These differences are properties of the physical structures involved in making stimulus-response connections.

The second postulate states how individuals can be grouped according to type. In an abbreviated form it is:

> Individuals in whom excitatory potential is generated slowly and in whom excitatory potentials so generated are relatively weak are predisposed to

develop extraverted patterns of behaviour; individuals in whom excitatory potential is generated quickly and in whom excitatory potentials so generated are strong, are predisposed to develop introverted patterns of behaviour.

In view of Eysenck's apparent assumption that excitation and inhibition are reciprocal or mutally exclusive, this second postulate is reiterated in converse form with the addition of concept of speed of dissipation:

> Similarly, individuals in whom reactive inhibition is developed quickly, in whom strong reactive inhibitions are generated, and in whom reactive inhibition is dissipated slowly, are predisposed to develop extraverted patterns of behaviour; conversely, individuals in whom reactive inhibition is developed slowly, in whom weak reactive inhibitions are generated, and in whom reactive inhibition is dissipated quickly, are predisposed to develop introverted patterns of behaviour.

In fact, the assumption that excitation and inhibition are reciprocal or mutally exclusive can be challenged since one can conceive of *two independent* neural systems, one inhibitory and one facilitatery, that can be independently excited, it being the *relative* extent of activation of the two systems that defines overall degree of excitation or inhibition (see the later discussion of Equilibrium of the nervous system, or Gray, 1970). If we further challenge two more assump-

Fig. 2.1 Types of individuals as defined by certain aspects of excitation and inhibition (I = introvert cell, E = extravert cell)

	Develops	Strength	Dissipates	Excitation			
				Develops FAST		Develops SLOW	
				STRONG	WEAK	STRONG	WEAK
INHIBITION	FAST	HIGH	FAST				
			SLOW				E
		LOW	FAST				
			SLOW				
	SLOW	HIGH	FAST				
			SLOW				
		LOW	FAST	I			
			SLOW				

tions — that a quickly (slowly) developed potential will be strong (weak), and that a quickly (slowly) developed inhibitory potential will dissipate slowly (quickly) — on the basis of a lack of explicity stated empirical evidence, then rather a complex pattern of possible personality types emerges (see Fig. 2.1) consists of 32 potential cells of which Eysenck's theory fills only two. Eysenck's theory can therefore be seen as a simplified version of this matrix, formed by collapsing cells together (see Fig. 2.2).

Even a cursory glance at the details of Eysenck's theory, however, reveals that despite the impression gleaned from the two postulates, he obviously does differentiate excitation and inhibition as more than just the two sides of the same coin. For example, he notes that 'Excitatory and inhibitory changes obey different laws; thus inhibition quickly dissipates with time, whereas excitation does not (1957, p. 46)'. In fact, on the whole, excitatory and inhibitory potentials are described as quite distinct systems. Excitation concerns the ease with which impulses can travel from neuron to neuron in a very general sense (and hence is easily linked with the non-specific facilitative effects on neural transmission of activation in the ascending reticular formation). But it also includes the growth of facilitatory connections between specific neurons (learning).

The definition of inhibition is rather more complex because of the extensive history of the term. Most typically we have, first, the external and internal distinction made by Pavlov (i.e. distraction by an external source v. an internal, gradual build-up of resistance to a conditioned reflex, such as in the extinction paradigm), which may be roughly aligned with spatial and temporal inhibition (distraction v. fatigue). Secondly, there are Hull's concepts of reactive inhibition

Fig. 2.2 Simplification of Fig. 2.1, Eysenck's model

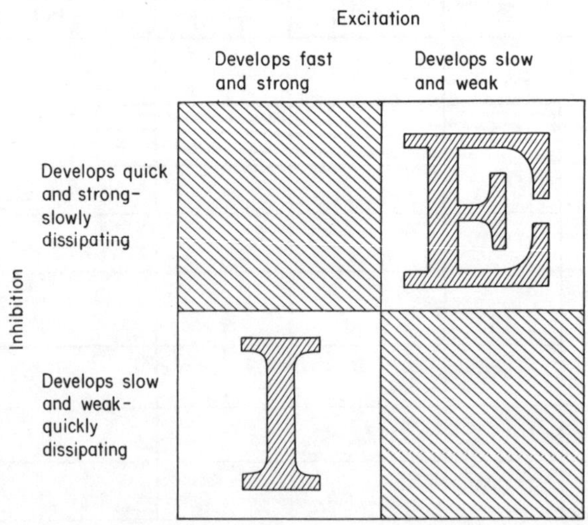

(I_R) and conditioned inhibition ($_SI_R$) (a type of neural fatigue v. a behavioural habit of not responding). However, Eysenck prudently avoids linking himself with any one precise theoretical definition of either excitation or inhibition, preferring an operational approach whereby these two processes are inferred from changes in the performance of subjects under specified experimental paradigms. For example, the acquisition of a conditioned eye-blink response is taken as an obvious facilitatory or excitatory process whereas its extinction would be an inhibitory phenomenon, as would be taking a rest pause during a boring task.

Evidence linking personality with cortical excitation and inhibition

In the *Dynamics of Anxiety and Hysteria* and *Biological Basis of Personality*, Eysenck (1957, 1967) summarises extensive evidence from many different experimental areas in support of his two basic postulates. No attempt will be made here to repeat such a review, but we shall consider those areas in which we have a better understanding of the neural correlates. Many of the areas that Eysenck examines, for example, may make reference to performance behaviours that are readily interpretable in terms of excitation and inhibition, but are still very woolly in terms of actual neural representation. This is, of course, a direct consequence of the fact that excitation and inhibition are 'hypothetical constructs . . . which cannot in their very nature be specifically located in any physiological structure (Eysenck, 1967, p. 81)'.

Despite this, if we stick to criterion behaviours that not only have reference to excitation and inhibition but are also more directly linked to brain structure and function, then we can more accurately relate personality to brain. Therefore, the areas of conditioning (Franks, 1954, 1956, 1957; Eysenck, 1965), reminiscence (Treadwell, 1956; Eysenck and Frith, 1977), work decrement (Broadbent, 1956; Claridge, 1956), homeostatic behaviour (Davis, 1949; Venables 1956), stress response (Venables, 1953, 1955), involuntary rest pauses (Franks, 1963; Eysenck, 1964), vigilance (Claridge, 1960; Bakan et al., 1963), stimulus-seeking (Weisen, 1965), persistence (Costello and Eysenck, 1966) and learning (Skanthakumari, 1965; Gebhart, 1966) will be merely summarised in Table 2.1. Further discussion will be limited to the effects of drugs which cross the blood-brain barriers (see also the discussion by Stelmack (1979) of certain psychophysiological measures such as the orientating reflex). This area is of central importance because it pertains most directly to a third postulate of Eysenck's theory that formally proposes that extraverts are generally less aroused than introverts:

> Depressant drugs increase cortical inhibition, decrease cortical excitation and thereby produce extraverted behaviour patterns. Stimulant drugs decrease cortical inhibition, increase cortical excitation and thereby produce introverted behaviour patterns. (Eysenck 1957, p. 229).

Table 2.1

Evidence relating extraversion-introversion to excitation-inhibition

Area	Theoretical relations to excitation — inhibition	Predicted performance	Supporting papers (examples)
1 Conditioning	Excitation facilitates conditioning	Extraverts condition poorly	Franks (1954, 1956, 1957) Jawanda (1966)
2 Reminisence	Rest pause allows inhibition to dissipate	Extraverts show more reminiscence	Treadwell (1956) Eysenck (1957)
3 Work decrement	A direct consequence of accumulating inhibition	Extraverts' work deteriorates quicker	Broadbent (1956) Furneaux (1955)
4 Homeostasis	Weak inhibition leads to over-reaction	Introverts over-compensate	Davis (1946, 1948, 1949) Veneables (1956)
5 CFF (critical flicker fusion)	Flickers fuse when previous after-image is not inhibited	Extraverts can see flicker at higher frequency	Krugman (1947) Goldstone (1955) Spielmann (1963)
6 Involuntary rest pauses	Pause due to inhibition build-up	Extraverts pause more frequently	Eysenck (1964) Franks (1963)
7 Vigilance	Inhibition causes loss of vigilance	Extraverts less vigilant	Bartenwerfer (1957) Hogan (1966)
8 Sensory thresholds	Higher excitation means greater sensitivity	Extraverts have higher thresholds	Smith (1966) Dunstone et al. (1964)
9 Pain threshold	Pain feeling can be inhibited	Extraverts can tolerate pain better	Lynn and Eysenck (1961) Haslam (1966)
10 Effector output	Excitation leads to greater effector response	Introverts respond (salivate) more to lemon juice	Corcoran (1964)
11 Learning	(a) Inhibition builds up in rote learning	Extraverts poorer at rote learning	Jensen (1964)
	(b) Interference has to be inhibited	Introverts react worse to distraction	Shanmugam and Santhanam (1964)
12 Spiral after-effects	After-effect stops due to inhibition	Extraverts show less after-effects	Lynn (1960) Holland (1965)

In assessing the available evidence pertaining to this drug postulate (see Table 2.2 for a summary of such evidence), Eysenck (1957) reaches several conclusions. First, many areas give relatively unambiguous evidence in favour of the drug postulate, in that the depressant drug shifts performance in the direction of extraverted behaviour. Second, the evidence in some other areas is difficult to evaluate since clear predictions of drug effects cannot be made because the nature of the task and its relation to inhibition/excitation (and hence personality) is ambiguous and obscure. Third, more detailed elaboration of the theory is extremely difficult at the moment because of frequently found curvilinear relationships between drug dose and performance effect (often interpretable as a manifestation of the Yerkes-Dodson law). Fourth, the prevalence of curvilinear associations is further complicated by personality interactions with drug effect (e.g. introverts, being more cortically excited, need a smaller stimulant dose to be pushed past the point of optimum performance). Fifth, groups of subjects in experiments do not generally have their other personality characteristics

Table 2.2
Summary of drug effects linking personality to excitation-inhibition

Task	Effect of stimulant	Effect of depressant	Effect of personality	Author
1 Sedation threshold	Moves S away from sedation	S is sedated	Extraverts (Es) readily sedated	Shagass (1954, 1955, 1956)
2 Reminiscence	Reduced	Increased	Higher in Es	Steinberg and Summerfield (1955)
3 Satiation	Decreased	Increased	Higher in Es	Bender (1952)
4 Vigilance	Improved	Decreased	Lower in Es	Mackworth (1948)
5 Spiral after-effects	Prolongs after-effect	Decreases after-effect	Shorter in Es	Eysenck (1957)
6 Work decrement	Delays decrement	Enhances decrement	More evident in Es	Eysenck (1957)
7 Visual masking (Bidwell)	Raises threshold (decreases) masking)	Lowers threshold (increases masking)	Lowers threshold in Es	Eysenck (1957)
8 Visual masking	Decreases	Increases	Increased in Es	Holland (1963)
9 Electrodermal conditioning	Increase autonomic conditioning	Decreased conditioning	Es show poorer conditioning	Jones et al. (1965)
10 Eyelid conditioning	Improves conditioning	Decreases conditioning	Poor in Es	Franks and Trouton (1958)
11 Verbal conditioning	Improves conditioning	Decreases conditioning	Poor in Es	Jawanda (1966)
12 Kinaesthetic figural after-effects	Smaller	Larger	Larger in Es	Gupta and Kaur (1978)
13 Contingent negative variation	Decrease in CNV	Increase in CNV	CNV enhanced in Es	Janssen et al. (1978)

matched, e.g. interactions between *E* and *N* should be anticipated.

An example of the difficulties in elucidating the complicated relationships between drugs, performance and personality is the work of Gupta (1974; Gupta and Singh, 1971; Gupta and Kaur, 1978). Gupta (1974) showed that the kinaesthetic figural after-effect (KFAE) was enhanced by 100 mg of phenobarbitone and reduced by 10 mg of dexedrine. This is in line with Eysenckien theory, but Gypta *failed* to find an interaction between drug effect and personality, which might have been predicted on the assumption that introverts and extraverts begin the study at different points on the arousal continuum.

Therefore, Gupta and Kaur (1978) undertook a carefully designed study to obtain, for the first time, dose-response data for the effect of 7.5, 10.0 and 12.5 mg of dextroamphetamine on KFAE, in groups of subjects of differing E-score. Three groups of *S*s were used: E^+ (14+), E (10 to 12) and E— (8—); and the groups were matched for N by rejecting all *S*s with N-scores more than one s.d. from the mean. The response surface is given in Fig. 2.3, including the data for the placebo (P) condition. It should be noted that height of the response surface indicates magnitude of KFAE response. It can be seen from Fig. 2.3, and verified statistically by Gupta, that (a) there is an interaction between personality and drug treatment ($p<.01$), (b) the extraverts (E^+) have higher KFAE scores than introverts (E—) under placebo conditions, as predicted by Eysenck, (c) the drug reduces the magnitude of KFAE in the E^+ group ($p< .01$ for each drug level), which is in line with Eysenck's predictions, (d) the drug increases the

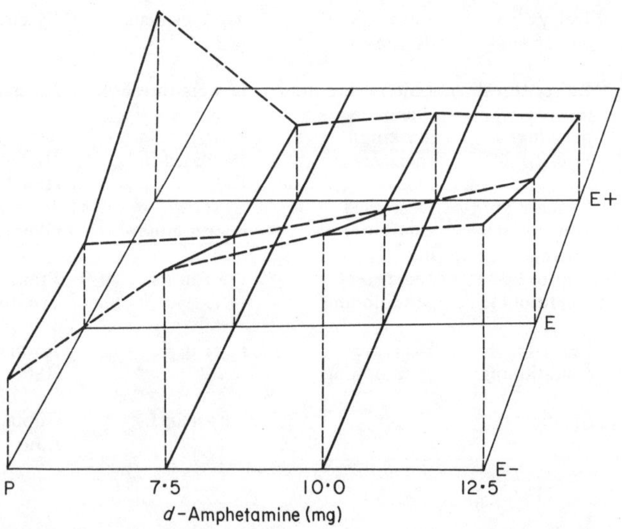

Fig. 2.3 Response surface: personality and drug treatments on kinaesthetic figural after-effects (from Gupre and Kaur, 1978)

magnitude of KFAE in the E$^-$ group ($p < .05$ for 7.5 mg does, $p < .01$ for both 10.0 and 12.5 mg dose), which can be explained by combining Eysenck's theory with the Yerkes-Dodson law.

One can conveniently summarise these findings by saying that 'the drug thus facilitates the judging capacity of extraverts but debilitates that of introverts'. That is to say, dextroamphetamine acts on the under-aroused cortex of the extravert to raise arousal so that performance can be more efficient (i.e. KFAE's smaller) whereas the introvert, who is already quite aroused cortically, is over-stimulated by the drug, past the level of optimum performance, and performance therefore drops (i.e. KFAE's larger).

This study demonstrates how carefully designed a study must be to yield meaningful results, for the same drug can at different doses both increase and decrease KFAE, and the same drug dose can, in two differing populations, cause opposing KFAE effects.

A further series of drug studies that are relevant to Eysenck's theory concern the treatment of hyperkinetic children with stimulant drugs. It can be noted beforehand that stimulant drugs generally improve the performance of normal children by raising cortical arousal to a more efficient level. These findings have been reviewed by Aman (1978) and are presented in Table 2.3 where the results for the three major stimulants used (methylphenidate, dextroamphetamine and deanol) are given separately. It can be seen that not all the stimulants need have identical effects, but that in general the direction of performance change is in the introverted direction. This is particularly true of those well-known tests of extraversion, the continuous performance test (greatly affected by the poor vigilance of the extraverts) and the Porteus maze test (where the extravert's impulsive tendency to go up blind alleys leads to greater error scores)

In spite of the fact that hyperactive children seem over-stimulated, at least behaviourally, stimulants have effects essentially identical to those found with normal children. For example, Barkley (1977) reviewed the literature to find that 74 per cent of 915 hyperactive children had a reduced attention deficit with amphetamine treatment; methylphenidate achieved a 77 per cent improvement across 866 children; and on 105 children magnesium pemoline achieved a 73 per cent improvement rate. These rates can be compared with a 39 per cent improvement rate for placebo conditions across 417 subjects.

The results of these studies are summarised in Table 2.4. In another review of the effects of stimulants on hyperactive and conduct disorders, Cantwell and Carlson (1978) make the point that it is more than just cognitive performance that is changed in an introverted direction, for gross behaviour, too, changes in a socialised (i.e. introverted) direction. As Cantwell and Carlson put it: 'the most consistant positive effect of the stimulants (other than caffeine and deanol) is on behaviour, particularly of the type perceived by teachers as disruptive and not socially appropriate'. They further point out that the personality change can be so dramatic as to disturb the child's relationship with parents: 'He's not my

Table 2.3
The effect of stimulants on cognitive performance in normal children (from Aman, 1978)

Task	Stimulant		
	Methyl-phenidate	Dextro-amphetamine	Deanol
1 Continuous performance tests	Improved	Improved	Improved
2 Reaction time	Improved		
3 Paired associate learning	Improved		
4 Matching familiar figures:			
(a) impulsivity	Improved		
(b) accuracy	Possible improvement	no change	no change
5 Verbal IQ	Possible improvement	Possible improvement	no change
6 Performance IQ	Improved	Improved	Improved
7 Bender Gestalt	Some improvement	no change	no change
8 Frosting test of visual perception	Some improvement	Possible improvement	
9 Illinois test of psycholinguistic ability (ITPA)	Improved		no change
10 Wepman test of auditory discrimination	no change	no change	
11 Porteus mazes	Improved	Improved	

child', 'He's a different boy', 'I don't have the same boy I used to', sometimes to the extent that they ask for medication to be discontinued.

The fact that stimulant drugs cause such an improvement suggests that the hyperactive child has an under-aroused cortex (i.e. in an extreme extravert-like state). Evidence for this proposition comes mainly from the laboratory of Satterfield (1973, 1978; Satterfield and Dawson, 1971; Satterfield et al., 1972, 1974). In their first study, Satterfield and Dawson (1971) found that 24 hyperactive children, matched to normal controls, had a low resting skin conductance level, a low frequency of non-specific skin conductance fluctuations and low amplitudes of skin conductance responses.

In a follow-up study, Satterfield et al. (1972) compared in 14 hyperactive children those who responded well to stimulant (methylphenidate) medication with those who responded poorly (*n*s of 6 and 5 respectively). The former group did indeed have lower CNS arousal as indicated by lower skin conductance levels,

Table 2.4
The effects of stimulants on the performance of hyperactive children

Task	Stimulant effect	Authors (examples)
1 Attention (CPT and RT)	Improved	Cohen et al. (1971), Werry and Aman (1975), Yepes et al. (1977)
2 Choice-RT	Improved	Reichardt and Elder (1978)
3 Cognitive style (MFF)	Improved impulsivity	Campbell et al. (1971)
4 WISC	Mixed results; mildly facilitative	Rapoport et al. (1974), Weiss et al. (1975), Hoffman et al. (1974), Weiss et al. (1971)
5 Bender Gestalt	No effect	Friedman et al. (1973), Garfinkel et al. (1975)
6 ITPA	Mixed results	Butter and Lapierre (1974, 1975), Douglas (1974)
7 Wepman test of auditory discrimination	No effect	Friedman et al. (1973), Weiss et al. (1971)
8 Porteus Maze	Improved	Connors et al. (1964), Gittelman-Klein and Klein (1976)
9 Lemon juice test	Increased response	McManis et al. (1978)

higher mean EEG amplitudes, more energy in the low-frequency bank of the EEG and larger auditory-evoked cortical potentials. In a similar vein, Satterfield et al. (1974) found that pre-treatment skin conductance levels correlated significantly ($r = .44$, $p < .05$, $n = 18$) with a good behavioural response to methylphenidate treatment. Further studies replicating these findings have been reviewed by Satterfield (1978) who goes on to postulate a model as to why low CNS arousal leads to the observed behaviours of poor vigilance, poor attention, impulsivity and so on.

Rather surprising, it is a low CNS arousal = low CNS inhibition model. I say surprising because most researchers would agree (e.g. Eysenck, 1967; Gray, 1967; Nebylitsyn, 1972) that the cortex is in an *inhibited* state when only lowly aroused. The relationship between CNS arousal, CNS excitation and CNS inhibition is made clear in Fig. 2.4; at low levels of CNS arousal there is a dominance of inhibitory potentials, at high levels a dominance of excitatory potentials, with a point in the middle (which probably coincides with the point of peak efficiency in the Yerkes-Dodson model) at which some balance is reached.

In reading Satterfield's model, however, it is clear that he has confused CNS inhibition with *behaviour* inhibition. The two are not synonymous and in fact are, if anything, reciprocal, for the overt behaviour of the low aroused extravert is uninhibited (e.g. tires of behaviours and tasks rapidly, prefers change, expansive and demonstrative gestures, impulsive) and the overt behaviour of the higher aroused introvert is generally inhibited (e.g. socially controlled, reflective and undemonstrative). But Satterfield has unwittingly placed emphasis on an important point, for poor vigilance, persistence and concentration and greater distractibility can be produced by a state of gross low inhibition, i.e. when the cortex is very aroused (this being the Yerkes-Dodson law again as reflected in Fig. 2.4).

This could lead one to hypothesise that there might be *two* groups (at least) of hyperactive children: first, those who are low aroused-high inhibited and who respond well to stimulant medication, and second, those who are high aroused-low inhibited and do not respond well to stimulant medication, and who may even worsen. The fact that only 60 to 70 per cent of hyperactive children respond well to stimulant drugs (Conners, 1972) suggests this might be the case: two groups of widely different CNS pathology are being grouped together on the basis of similar overt behaviour pathology. The obvious question to ask is whether the second, postulated over-aroused group would respond well to depressant medication. Unfortunately this study has not been done, so far as the author is aware. However, there is a group of children who have much in common behaviourally with hyperkinetic children who *are* treated by a sedating drug — those with tics and Tourette's syndrome.

In a review of the literature on tics, Corbett (1977) points out that 'although the tic syndrome does not "crystallise" before the sixth or seventh year of life, in most patients there have been previous behavioural symptoms, either in the form of hyperkinesis, dyskinesia or impulsiveness', and that overactive behaviour has been reported in many cases. In addition, there is a preponderance of boys in the ratio of about 3:1, as with the hyperactive syndrome. Ticqueurs, who

Fig. 2.4 The relationship between arousal, excitation and inhibition in the CNS

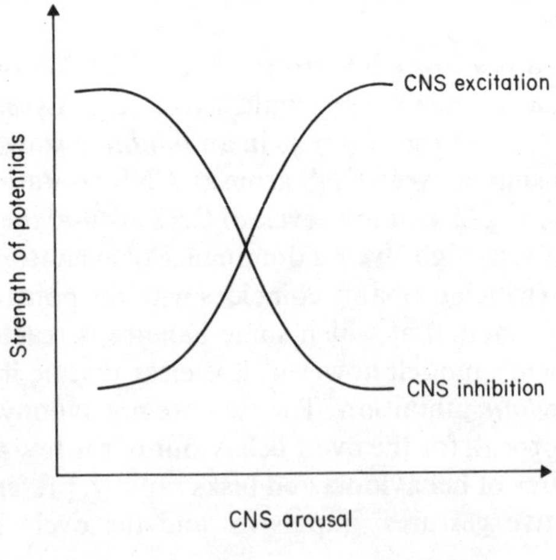

show distinct elements of hyperactivity as just described, are treated not with stimulants but mainly with haloperidol (see Corbett, 1977, for a discussion of the various drugs used). Haloperidol, although essentially an antipsychotic, is also a sedative and depresses the activity of the brain stem (Winsberg and Yepes, 1978).

It is convenient at this point to fill in the last details of Eysenck's theory, which, as has already been mentioned briefly, concerns the identification of arousal, excitation and inhibition with the functioning of the brain-stem reticular formation (the ascending reticular activating system) and the visceral brain (hippocampus, amygdala, cingulum, septum and hypothalamus). The theory is best stated in Eysenck's (1967) own words, which can be related to the diagrammatic representation in Fig. 2.5:

> We have two sets of loops, which are in turn connected with each other. The first of these is the cortico-reticular loop. Neural messages ('sensations') going along the classical ascending pathways relay to the particular projection areas involved in the cortex; they also send collaterals into the reticular formation, which in turn sends 'arousal' messages to the cortex to keep it in a state of functional tonus. Depending on the nature of the infor-

Fig. 2.5 Diagrammatic representation of mutual interaction of reticular formation, visceral brain, and cortex. Direct arousing effects of visceral brain stimulation are not indicated in this figure

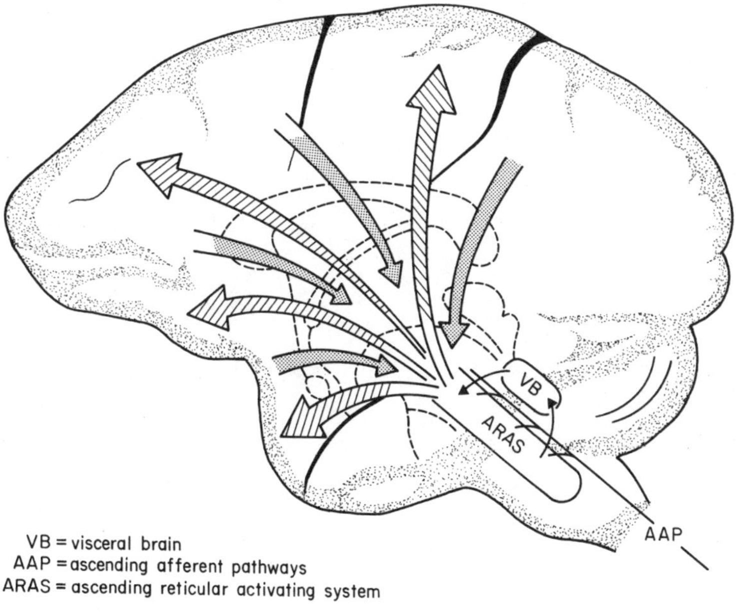

mation transmitted, the cortex in turn instructs the reticular formation to continue sending 'arousal' messages or else to switch to 'inhibition'. *This loop then is concerned with information processing, with cortical arousal and inhibition, and in its application to personality differences with introversion and extraversion.*

The second loop concerns the visceral brain and the reticular formation. Messages from the visceral brain also reach the reticular formation via collaterals and having arousing effects on the cortex in a manner very similar to that produced by information received via the ascending afferent pathways. *It is this loop that is concerned with emotion, and in its application to personality differences, with neuroticism/emotionality* (pp. 231-2, my italics).

Evidence in favour of the importance of the first, corticoreticular, loop for personality obviously comes from the accuracy of the drug postulate, since stimulants and depressants act directly on reticular activity. This evidence has already been discussed (see Tables 2.2-2.4).

Evidence in favour of the importance of the second, visceral brain loop will be discussed later when the effects of lesions in the limbic system and in Papez's circuit are reviewed.

3 Some modifications to Eysenck's theory: Gray's model

There have been many criticisms of Eysenck's theory, inevitably, given its extreme breadth of coverage and its foundation on, in many areas, rather sketchy evidence. Indeed, Eysenck (1967) in his epilogue to *Biological Basis of Personality* has no doubts that it is a 'weak' theory, useful primarily for the guidance of future research. In this spirit, we shall not deal here with minor criticisms of specific studies, but with broader questions that (a) promise to clarify or extend or augment the theory as a whole, (b) more directly concern the brain, given the context of the present book.

For these reasons, topics such as whether hysterics and dysthymics are really suitable criterion groups for experiments, or whether incarcerated prisoners can respond to the extraversion questionnaire scale with any validity, will be foregone.

The first point of discussion concerns the manner in which excitation and inhibition are measured — or, rather, not measured. As Eysenck (1967) clearly says, it is essential for his full theory that both excitatory and inhibitory processes or potentials should be assessed independently — 'Ideally, no doubt, one would like to measure both excitatory and inhibitory potentials separately (p. 80)' — before the full power of the theory can be reached. For example, although Eysenck sees differences in the accumulation of inhibition as most important for predicting eye-blink conditioning, certain anomalous results lead him to suggest 'that differences in excitation may not be negligible, even though they may be less important than differences in inhibition (p. 120)'.

In fact there is little point in postulating dual processes if there is no way of individually evaluating them. If they always move in an inextricably linked and constant manner then it would be more parsimonious to phrase the theory totally in one-factor terms, which would reduce the model to a simple arousal theory (of the kind so far used to explain many other sets of behaviours including schizophrenia and autism) and make any kind of elegant prediction impossible. Logically, it should not be necessary to have this state of affairs forced upon the theory, since if it is essential to posit both processes in order to explain individual differences on particular tasks and to account for various phenomena, then it would imply that a knowledge of an individual performance at these tasks should in some way describe the functioning of both his excitatory and inhibitory circuits. For example, some tasks could be said to measure mainly excitatory effects (e.g. speed of acquisition of a conditioned response (CR), sensory thresholds, effector response) and others mainly inhibitory effects (e.g. work decrement, habituation rate, involuntary rest pauses, rate of extinction of CR, vigilance). We need, therefore, to test individuals on a series or battery of tests that relate to differing aspects of excitation and inhibition, and link the resultant pattern to extraversion scores, rather than, as is done at present, relate E-scores to a single criterion task that might involve many other aspects of processing tangential to the theory. The latter approach can only serve to underestimate the power of the theory.

We can adapt Fig. 2.1 to provide a more refined set of predictions of E on the basis of task preformance. This adaptation is shown in Fig. 3.1, where each cell scores +1 point every time it coincides with an extraverted (+) branch of the theory, and —1 for each time it coincides with an introverted (—) branch. The scores range from the pure introvert at —5 to the pure extravert at +5, with ambiverts of various value in between.

Further progress of Eysenck's theory may well depend, then, on the ability of the experimenter to devise ways of separately measuring the different facets of both excitation and inhibition, with a view to building up a picture of the individual's pattern of functioning, so as to better predict other aspects of the subject's experimental, personal and social behaviour. The theory could then begin to

Fig. 3.1 Hypothetical relationship between the performance of inhibitory and excitatory potentials and extraversion (see text for explanation). The scores range from +5 (extreme extravert) to —5 (extreme introvert)

					Excitation			
					Develops Fast (—)		Develops Slow (+)	
					Strong (—)	Weak (+)	Strong (—)	Weak (+)
INHIBITION	FAST (+)	HIGH	(+)	Fast (—)	—1	+1	+1	+3
				Slow (+)	+1	+3	+3	+5
		LOW	(—)	Fast (—)	—3	—1	—1	+1
				Slow (+)	—1	+1	+1	+3
	SLOW (—)	HIGH	(+)	Fast (—)	—3	—1	—1	+1
				Slow (+)	—1	+1	+1	+3
		LOW	(—)	Fast (—)	—5	—3	—3	—1
				Slow (+)	—3	—1	—1	+1

operate better at the individual person level rather than, as is the case now, at the general group level. This is a direction of movement identical with other areas of neuropsychology, where, for example, it may be known that in general right-handers have speech in the left hemisphere, but that a simple, specific test of *degree* of lateralisation (such as supplied by tachistoscopic procedures) will better predict an individual's reaction to circumstances such as brain surgery, lesions and recovery from aphasia (Buffery, 1977).

The second point of discussion regarding the modification of Eysenck's theory emanates from the work of Gray (1970, 1972) who makes an important point concerning conditionability, which then has ramifications for the physiological substrate.

The initial stage in Gray's argument is to suggest that the socialised behaviour of the introvert cannot be properly accounted for by the blanket reason 'because they are better at conditioning', since the introvert conditions better than the extravert *only under certain circumstances*, such as when partial reinforcement is used, with weak CSs and USs, and with short CS-UCS intervals (see Mangan 1974, for a similar discussion). For instance, in the eye-blink conditioning study by Eysenck and Levey (1967) it was the use of a low-intensity puff of air and a shorter CS-UCS interval that favoured the introvert. Given these particular constraints on superior introvert conditioning, the argument is that we have no particular reason to suppose that these criteria are more likely to be met during development than any other set of conditions. Why, then, does the introvert end up looking more conditioned?

Gray's postulate is that introverts and extroverts do not differ in the ability to be conditioned *per se*, but differ in their susceptibility to punishment and fear, so that the introvert's superior conditioning depends on the degree of threat encountered. He points out that psychopaths (high E) behave with no apparent thought of punishment consequences whereas dysthymics (high I) are extremely fearful people. This analysis does not conflict with the interpretation of conditioning phenomena in terms of arousal put forward by Eysenck (1965), Corcoran (1964) and Spence (1964), for it can be claimed that the more aroused an individual is, the quicker a stimulus becomes a punisher (in the same way, perhaps, that the pain threshold is reached more quickly in a more aroused person).

At this point, it could be queried whether Gray's modification represents any advance upon Eysenck's original theory: simply, can it be claimed that socialisation and development proceed primarily contingent upon negative, punishment learning experiences, with any greater validity than the conditionability thesis? Gray does not take up this issue, and indeed objective evidence is difficult to muster, but one of the most careful and thorough theoretical analyses of the basis of social behaviour, Kelvin (1974) can be instructive. Kelvin reasons that implicit, unstated, interpersonal expectations control our behaviour; that we proceed in accord with that which is expected of us. Social pressure, and forces to conformity, are only exerted when unexpected behaviour is emitted. We are not, therefore, aware of external contingencies until a deviant act is committed, and we are 'rewarded' for normalised behaviour only in the sense that it avoids the experience of controlling forces. This is a pretty clear statement of avoidance and punishment paradigms of the type that the introvert is most susceptible to according to Gray's theory.

To return to the body of Gray's theory, the conceptualisation of the introvert as more susceptible to punishment precipitates a reworking of the physiological theory. What is the neural substrate of this mechanism? It starts with the recognition of two basic 'facts' — (a) barbiturates have extraverting effects, (b) frontal lesions have extraverting effects — and one basic assumption: if we better understand the nature of the action of barbiturates and frontal lesions then we will have a better understanding of the basis of extraversion.

Summarising Gray's (1972) article, we proceed as follows

1 Barbiturates antagonise the activity of the punishment mechanism: sodium amobarbital reduces passive avoidance in rats (Miller, 1959) and also the effects of frustrative non-reward (Amsel, 1962), while simple approach learning to a positive reinforcer remains unimpaired. (Kamano et al. 1966).

2 Barbiturates have the same action as lesions in the limbic system. Although the major action of sodium amobarbital is on the ARAS, this cannot account for the drug's effect of differential sensitivity to punishment. The secondary action of the drug is upon the limbic system; more particularly, on the hippocampus and those cells in the medial septal area that act as the pacemaker for hippocampal theta (Stumpf, 1965). Driving or blocking the theta rhythm changes speed of and resistance to extinction, as does sodium amobarbital, i.e. lesioning that causes theta-blocking leads to rapid extinction.

3 Lesions in the orbital front cortex have the same action as barbiturates and lesions in the limbic system. Frontal lesions impair passive avoidance learning (Grossman, 1967) and specifically *orbital* lesions have effects in rhesus monkeys very similar to lesions in the medial septal area (Butters and Rosvold, 1968). Here, it should be noted that the orbital frontal cortex is the highest controlling area for the septohippocampal system.

Hence a system has been described consisting of the orbital frontal cortex, the medial septal area and the hippocampus, in which high activity will mimic the sensitivity to punishment of the introvert. This system will operate in conjunction with the ARAS because the pacemaker cells in the medial septal region that drive hippocampal theta are themselves activated by input from the midbrain reticular formation. Further, activity in the ARAS is itself depressed by hippocampal theta activity, thus creating a negative feedback loop, whereby increased ARAS activity increases hippocampal activity that inhibits ARAS activity. The whole scheme can now be diagrammatically represented in Fig. 3.2. It can be seen that there are two basic differences to Eysenck's corticoreticular loop model: the cortical aspect is restricted to the specific region of the orbital frontal

Fig. 3.2 The physiological basis of extraversion, Gray's theory (from Gray, 1972)

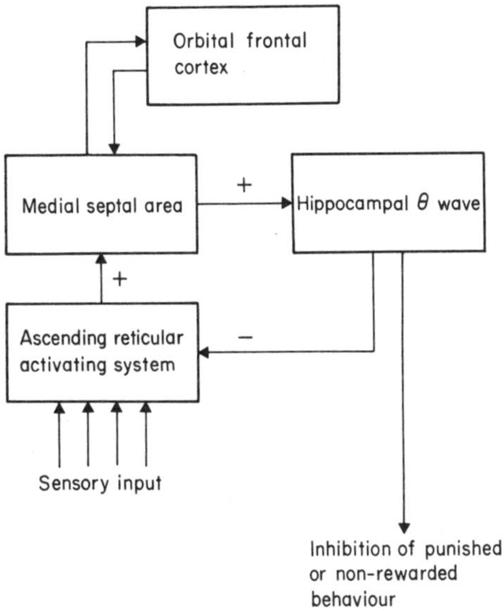

cortex; the limbic system is introduced into the corticoreticular loop, whereas Eysenck considers it somewhat separately, as underlying the neurotic dimension of personality.

Naturally enough, Gray's model has a few problems of its own. They might be outlined as follows

1 There is no direct evidence that socialisation proceeds through punishment contingencies - a point that has been raised already.
2 There is no direct evidence that introverts are more sensitive to punishment and frustrative non-rewards than are extraverts. Such evidence as there is comes from a *posthoc* analysis of studies designed to test other hypotheses. The *post-hoc* assessment of the 'degree of threat' imposed by various experimental procedures can only be very difficult. New studies need carrying out that will systematically vary this parameter and include positive reinforcement conditions.
3 The model is really an animal analogue, with no guarantee of its generalisability to humans. Until an animal study shows that language is primarily on the left in humans, I will remain cautious of animal studies that relate to human neuropsychological characteristics. The two human frontal lobes, for instance, are differentially involved in verbal tasks (Drewe, 1976).
4 There is no evidence that, in humans, the orbital frontal cortex is especially

linked to extraversion (remembering that Eysenck considers that cortical damage will in general have extraverting effects). Without wishing to pre-empt the later review of the effects of frontal lesions, it might be mentioned that in their study of leucotomised patients, Meyer and Beck (1954) equate personality change more with lesions to the dorsolateral and lateral cortex, whereas the orbito-insulo-temporo-cingulate complex is linked with emotional expression and experience (see also Fulton, 1951). Hence lesions in this latter system may reduce neuroticism and anxiety scores significantly but leave extraversion scores unaffected (Kelly, 1973). Russian neuropsychologists such as Homskaya (1973) also seem to accept that orbitofrontal lesions lead mainly to emotional disturbances. As a further example, Levinson and Meyer (1965) tested 29 patients before and after orbital undercutting, and found an immediate and highly significant change in neuroticism and manifest anxiety, but no similar change in extraversion.

Finally, it has to be made explicit that Gray's theory pertains both to Extraversion *and* Neuroticism, since his circuit underlays a personality dimension running from the introverted-neurotic quadrant to the extraverted-stable quadrant. Therefore, frontal and cingulate gyrus lesions should both increase extraversion and decrease neuroticism. It will be seen that this latter aspect of Gray's theory receives the full support of the data.

4 Strength, mobility, dynamism and equilibrium of the nervous system: the Russian school

Whereas Eysenck's work began with a description and classification of individuals at the level of personal overt behaviour, and expanded both in more molar directions (i.e. socialisation) and more molecular directions (i.e. properties of the nervous system), Russian work as propounded by Pavlov, Teplov and Nebylitsyn begins with properties and types of nervous activity — and stays there. According to Teplov (1964) one is forced to analyse man using indices at the Pavlovian level since 'real life' indices are masked by the enormous sum of conditioned connections that have been built up from birth: actual current overt behaviour is an 'alloy' of (a) type of nervous system and (b) conditioning experiences. The Russian school describe four properties of the nervous system — strength, mobility, dynamism and equilibrium — which will be described in turn and then related to western theorising. Because their experimental techniques are in many case unfamiliar to us, they will be described in some detail.

Strong and weak nervous systems

A strong nervous system is that which can withstand long and concentrated excitation, or the action of an 'ultra-strong' stimulus, without passing into an inhibitory state. There are two possible explanations for weakness (Teplov, 1964); (a) a small supply of some excitatory substance, or (b) an excitatory substance that is easy to destruct functionally. The second is preferred because it predicts not only the wilting reaction to intense work but also the fact that the weak system is more sensitive or highly reactive, i.e. if the excitatory substance is easily broken down then a given stimulus will have a greater impact on the nervous system.

The experimental paradigm most clearly allied to the above definition concerns the law of strength, which states that a conditioned reflex will increase in magnitude with greater intensity stimuli, until a point of stimulus intensity is reached at which inhibitions will occur so that the CR will no longer increase in magnitude and may actually fall or cease altogether. This is known as the point or threshold of transmarginal inhibition, which will be reached sooner in a weak system. From the descriptions of Teplov it would seem that experimenters often have to go to extreme and ingenious lengths to produce ultra-strong stimulation. He recounts the case of one laboratory worker hurtling into the experimental room, towards a harnessed dog, whirling an especially loud rattle and dressed in sheepskin. In Fig. 4.1 we have the law of strength results from two dogs Vot-te

Fig. 4.1 The magnitude of the conditioned response as dependent upon the magnitude of conditioning stimulus, for two dogs

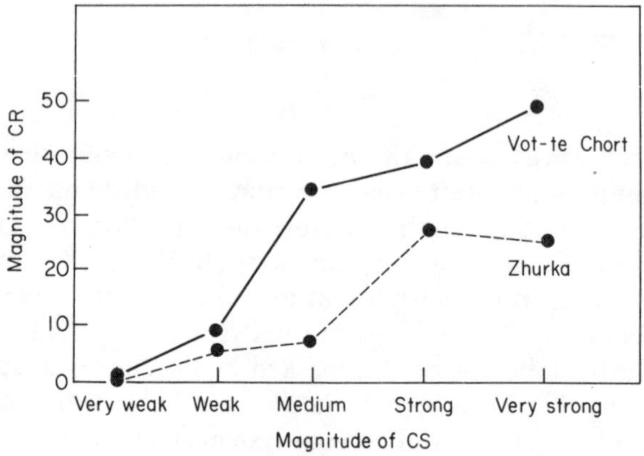

Chort and Zhurka. It can be seen that Zhurka has a weak nervous system, and Vot-te a strong one since he demonstrates the law of strength right up to the very strong stimulus.

Unfortunately, this assessment methodology that is basically simple and straightforward cannot be used with humans in its unadulterated form, because it is almost impossible to find in man the point at which the law of strength breaks down: we can tolerate stimuli of too great an intensity. Various alternatives are available, some of which involve the artificial heightening of the excitability in the cortical cells so that there is no need to use such extreme stimuli. For instance, the effects of caffeine can be observed: 'In the strong type a definite dose of caffeine increases the effect of the excitatory process; in the weak type it diminishes this effect causing the cell to overstep the limits of its working capacity (Pavlov, 1928)'. Caffeine increases excitability, thereby reducing working capacity, which makes the limit to the law of strength easier to find.

It can be seen, though, that this is a much more complicated method than the test on Vot-te and Zhurka, for it necessitates ascertaining the appropriate level of dosage of caffeine.

In man, there are at least five commonly used methods of measuring strength of the nervous system. These are most clearly described by Gray (1964).

Threshold of transmarginal (protective) inhibition

The two most frequently used experimental methods involve defining strength as the maximum time that a cell can work for when responding to a repeated stimulus. For obvious reasons, they are known as 'summation' methods — many small stimuli added together being regarded as having similar effects to one single ultra-strong stimulus. These two methods are the ergographic and photo-

Fig. 4.2 Hypothetical induction curves for a weak and strong nervous system

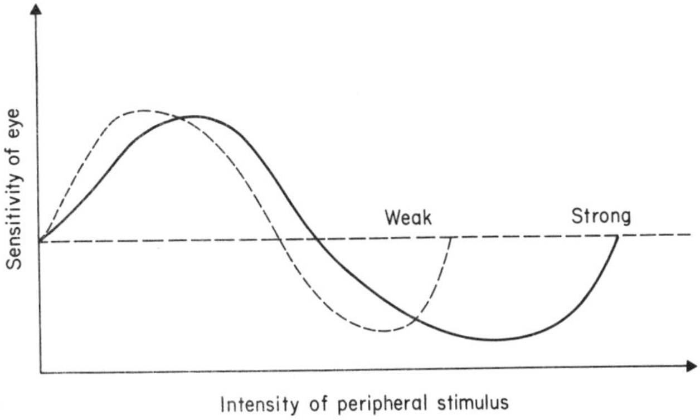

chemical conditioned reflex procedures. In the first, the response is to lift a weight attached to the middle finger after an auditory stimulus. A diminution of the response (i.e. lessened height of movement) after the administration of caffeine is taken as an indication of a weak system, for the caffeine is assumed to have taken the subject to the point of transmarginal inhibition (Rozhdestvenskaya, 1959). In the second, photochemical, method a conditioned response (photochemical conditioned reflex) is repeatedly elicited with reinforcement until the magnitude of the response declines. An early decrease will indicate a weak system and a late or absent decline a strong system (Rozhdestvenskaya, 1959).

Threshold of concentration and irradiation of excitation

The establishment of this threshold utilises what is known as the induction method. This is based on the phenomenon that the sensitivity of a dark-adapted eye to a point of light in peripheral vision is raised (improved) by a further weak point of light somewhere else in the periphery and lowered if the further point of light is strong — giving rise to the induction curve as in Fig. 4.2. The argument is that a strong system will withstand a higher degree of peripheral stimulation before sensitivity is adversely affected. The explanation of the phenomenon involves the idea that a weak stimulus will irradiate excitation over the cortex, initially facilitating the operation of other cortical areas.

Absolute sensory thresholds

Here, as mentioned previously, we would expect a negative correlation between strength of the nervous system and absolute sensory thresholds, as measured in the usual manner (Nebylitsyn et al. 1960).

Reaction time and stimulus intensity

If we plot the reaction time to stimuli of increasing intensity then the negative slope of the line (as in Fig. 4.3) is taken to be proportional to strength (Nebylitsyn, 1966; Zhorov and Yermolayeva-Tomina, 1972). The reason lies in the high excitability of the weak nervous system, for this 'allows it to respond at full speed at a point where for the strong, but less excitable, nervous system, the level of stimulation is not yet fully effective'.

Attention and distractibility

Here, the observation is that distracting stimuli cause the strong nervous system to concentrate harder, causing an improvement in performance and sensitivity, whereas the same distracting stimuli in a weak system will cause attention to break down so that performance and sensitivity suffer.

Strength of the nervous system and arousal theory

So far, the Russian model has had very little to do with 'brain' even though it is ostensibly a 'cortical' theory. The accent is very much on a description of human performance, with scant regard for actual neurophysiology or real brain structure. But, as with Eysenck's concepts of excitation and inhibition, strength of the nervous system is a hypothetical construct. Again, though, as with Eysenck's model, the hypothetical construct of strength can be linked with the concept of arousal - that has a quite well defined organic substrate. If we return to the five experimental paradigms described immediately above, then it can be seen that the results can easily be interpreted in terms of arousal theory.

(a) Transmarginal inhibition. The more aroused individual will, under condi-

Fig. 4.3 Hypothetical relationship between reaction time, stimulus intensity and strength of the nervous system

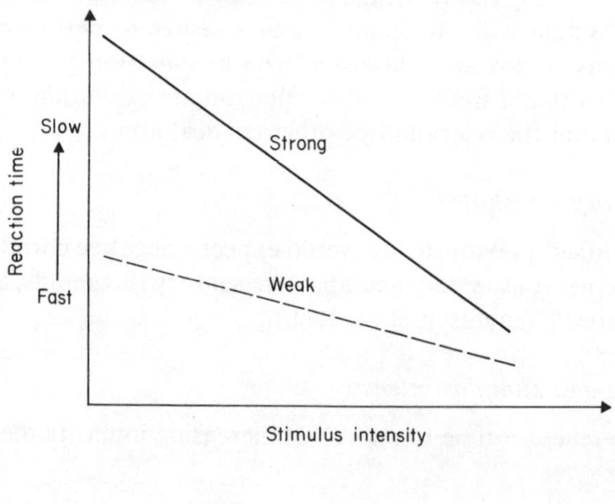

tions of gradually increasing arousal, pass the point of optimal performance on the Yerkes-Dodson curve sooner than the less aroused individual. Similarly, caffeine, being a stimulant, is more likely to cause an aroused individual to pass the optimum.

(b) Irradiation. Peripheral stimulation is more likely to improve the performance of a low aroused individual by increasing the arousal of the cortex, whereas in an already aroused individual, the extra stimulation caused by the peripheral stimulus is more likely to move the performance past the optimum.

(c) Sensory thresholds. An under-aroused, drowsy cortex is less likely to perceive very low level stimulation, while an alert, more aroused cortex is more likely to detect very weak stimuli.

(d) Reaction time. This is likely to be better when the cortex and organism is more aroused.

(e) Attention. Distraction is more likely to be detrimental to the already aroused cortex, by pushing arousal past the optimum level.

A much more detailed analysis of this kind has been made by Gray (1964), who makes the point that arousal theory (Malmo, 1959) and the law of strength can be written out in an identical format, such that predictions from the two models should be virtually identical:

> Arousal law: from low activation up to a point that is optimal for a given function, level of performance rises monotonically with increasing activation level . . . further increase in activation beyond this point produces a fall in performance level.
>
> Strength law: from low stimulus intensity up to a point that is optimal for a given function, response magnitude rises monotonically with increasing stimulus intensity . . . further increase in stimulus intensity beyond this point produces a fall in response magnitude.

Therefore, Gray develops the hypothesis that a weak nervous system is that which is in a more aroused state — whose cortex is bombarded non-specifically by the ARAS, as he puts it. Conversely, the strong system is generally in a less aroused state.

Strength of the nervous system and extraversion

If it is the weak nervous system that is more aroused, then it is tempting to equate the weak individual with the introvert, and the strong nervous system with the extravert: given, that is, Eysenck's theory relating extraversion to non-specific cortical arousal and neglecting, for the moment, Gray's modification. In one of the few Russian studies that use personality questionnaires, this hypothesis was specifically tested by Zhorov and Yermolayeva-Tomina (1972). In this study, 25 students (14 male, age range 18 to 25 years) completed forms A and B of the EPI, which had been translated into Russian. The measure of strength was the extent to which reaction time changed according to stimulus intensity, as described in Fig. 4.3. To this end, the subjects reacted to 1000 c/s tones at 10, 30, 50, 70 and 90 dB, after a 2 sec. visual warning signal. For each *S* a linear regression line was fitted to their performance, the slope of which (b, as in $y = a + bx$) was correlated with E-scores. Remembering that the extraverts should have strong nervous systems and large slopes, the actually obtained correlation between E and b was —.344; that is to say, nearly significant ($p < .10$) in the *wrong* direction. Similarly, when the nine most extraverted *S*s were compared with the eight most introverted ones, their mean slopes were 3.2 and 5.5 respectively, again contrary to prediction, and nearly significant so ($s <$!.1 on a *t*-test).

If we accept this result as valid, i.e. that it was a fair test of the hypothesis assuming that the Russian translation of the test is a viable procedure, then one is forced to reconsider the apparent nicety with which strength could be aligned with arousal as in the previous section. Gray (1967) points out that although experiments on sensory thresholds, distraction, transmarginal inhibition, flicker phenomena and drug effects do indicate some kind of correspondence between extraversion and strength, there is one notable area of disparity.

It is that extraverts have higher indices of EEG α-activity (Savage, 1964; Marton and Urban, 1966) — a high level of α being representative of low arousal — but that α-activity does not correlate with strength of the nervous system (Nebylitsyn, 1963, 1966). If these results continue to be replicated then we will be forced to conclude that although the law of strength and arousal theory make the same predictions on many tasks, they do so from a completely different vantage point, i.e. they concern separate aspects of central nervous system functioning. We must also conclude that both aspects are important or operational in the kinds of experimental paradigms so far cited. My hypothesis is that the simplest way of conceptualising these two separate but related aspects is to stick fairly closely to the original definitions of strength and arousal, perhaps as follows.

> Strength concerns the properties of neurons in terms of an 'excitability' substance that governs *working capacity.*
>
> Arousal concerns the triggering of neurons into degrees of activity by the ARAS in response to the *degree of workload.*

I think one can see that the concepts of work capacity and workload are by definition quite separate, one being an intrinsic quality of the nervous system, the other an extrinsic demand. But they are functionally highly related: in the way, for example, that 'having a low working capacity' and 'having a high workload' might be used interchangeably and both predict imminent exhaustion. With a few refinements, both of these definitions could be made to account for the known results, but only one of them, arousal, concerns the activity of the ARAS and such indices as α-activity.

Mobility of the nervous system

The dimension of mobility v. inertness is the second property of the nervous system and concentrates on the speed of adaptation of the organism to new circumstances.

> The mobility of the nervous process is defined by the speed at which they proceed, i.e. the speed with which they arise and then concentrate after the initial phase of irradiation, and also the speed of their disappearance when the stimulus has ceased to act. Another index of mobility is the speed with which one process is replaced by the opposing process. (Yakovleva, 1938)

These are, then, temporal aspects of nervous system and concern all aspects where the term 'speed' is appropriate (Teplov, 1964). Teplov describes various way to measure mobility including (a) the speed with which nervous processes terminate, such as the duration of the after-image, (b) the speed with which inhibition can change to excitation and vice versa, such as when a stimulus to perform is rapidly followed by a stimulus not to perform, (c) the speed of formation of conditioned associations, (d) rate of change in response to changes in external conditions as when an S^+ is changed to an S^-.

This dimension has no precise equivalent in western psychology. It pertains to some extent to Eysenck's 'conditionability' but only involves speed of CR acquisition and not its eventual strength; it does smack of heightened inhibition as in Eysenck's work with spiral and kinaesthetic after-effects, but then heightened excitation must be equally important because of the speed aspect.

There is little, then, to say about this dimension in the present context of personality and brain, since it has no special personality referent and no particular definition in terms of organic brain.

Dynamism of the nervous system

In contrast to the dimension of mobility, that seems to have little utility at present, dynamism would appear to be very germane indeed to western psychology because it is almost equivalent to the concept of conditionability — as originally put forward, say, by Eysenck before he refined his ideas and replaced this generalised notion with a specification of which conditions would favour conditioning in introverts.

As Gray (1967) describes, dynamism is the ability to form both positive conditioned reflexes and inhibitory conditioned reflexes (dynamism of the excitatory and inhibitory processes respectively). This twofold definition constitutes, in fact, something of a departure from Eysenck's theorising, since Eysenck — as noted in the previous sections — tends not to consider the separate measurement of positive and inhibitory conditioning. However, because Eysenck assumes that excitatory and inhibitory potentials and processes are reciprocal, then we would adduce that introverts, being considered as good, positive conditioners, would be poor inhibitory conditioners; or, in Russian terms, high on dynamism of excitatory processes and low on dynamism of inhibitory processes. We can now see that Eysenck's view of the excitation-inhibition balance is comparable to the idea of balance between the two types of dynamism. (This latter balance can be called equilibrium in dynamism where the term equilibrium is a fourth Russian dimension that describes the relative strength of excitatory and inhibitory processes in the three orthogonal dimensions of strength, mobility and dynamism; see Gray, 1967).

But, because Eysenck's ideas have 'moved on' to the extent that introverts are no longer seen as *always* better at conditioning — only with a weak UCS and short CS-UCS interval (Eysenck and Levey, 1966) — we cannot identify extraversion-introversion with equilibrium in dynamism. However, just because introverts are not conditionable across-the-board, does not mean that a dimension of generalised conditionability does not exist: only that Eysenck will not look for it because it no longer seems pertinent to his personality model.

The question of whether there exists a dimension of conditionability cannot be properly answered at the moment. That is, we cannot affirm whether individuals exist who condition well to both strong and weak UCSs with both long and short CS-UCSs and across many different types of CR. In western conditioning studies, subjects are never put through a whole battery of various types of conditioning experiences but are normally just tested under one paradigm with all task parameters held constant. The origin of dynamism suggests that Russian studies do exist that relate to this matter. But they remain, at present, still in Russian, untranslated.

5 Damagedness of the brain and personality

Both the Eysenkian and Pavlovian personality schemes are models in search of an organic basis. An alternative approach is to study the effects of damage to different areas of brain in the hope of perceiving patterns of relationships between the physical indices and behaviour. Both approaches are essential, in the way, for example, that our knowledge of memory has been advanced by laboratory studies of normals on the one hand and clinical observations of temporal, hippocampal and Korsakoff patients on the other. Ideally, the two types of inquiry stimulate and feed into each other so that a true neuropsychological model of memory would account for both laboratory and clinical phenomena. The same must hold true for other human facets such as language or, in this case, personality.

Damagedness of brain

The term damagedness will refer to the degree of brain injury as assessed by global measures (i.e. not pertaining to site of lesion), such as the depth of penetration of lesions, the number of lobes involved, the volume of tissue affected and extent of raised intracranial pressure.

Perhaps the most obvious example of generalised damage, is in the case of boxing. Each blow to the head causes neurons to die. As they do so, the brain shrinks, the ventricles expand, and the sulci on the cortex become more pronounced. There is a gradual intellectual deterioration and marked changes in personality are described, which may include apathy and loss of motivation and signs of loss of emotional control, evidenced by irritability and outbursts of temper (Roberts, 1969).

The first point to make is that a brain lesion is liable to have at least two effects: (a) effects attributable to the specific site of lesioning, such as loss of speech, paralysis or visual field defects, (b) general effects relating to the fact of having *any* brain malfunction or assault. In the same way a particular physical illness will have specific symptoms but most illnesses can cause degrees of distress, confusion, depression and lassitude.

Hécaen (1964) nicely demonstrates this difference between specific effects and damagedness effects, to reveal that both have implications for behaviours, cognitions and emotions that might pertain to personality. Hécaen initially describes how 94 individuals in a series of 439 tumour cases had mood and character changes and 161 showed confusion and cognitive deterioration. He then analyses the data with respect to both site of tumour and a general index of damagedness, the presence or absence of papilloedema, which indicates cranial hypertension of the type found with many kinds of brain damage. The results are given in Table 5.1, where it can be seen that confusional states are much more common if papilloedema is present ($p < .01$) and also most common in the specifically frontal group. The pattern is slightly more complex when it comes to personality changes, for although the last three groups indicate that personality change is more common with than without papilloedema, the trend is reversed for the frontals, who also have the highest rates of disturbance. Broadly speaking, we can say that damage to the brain, especially if it has a generalised effect as indicated by the presence of papilloedema, leads to a deterioration of cognitive processing and changes in mood and character. This general effect of damagedness is enhanced if the tumour is specifically in the front region.

It is a far cry, however, from saying that damagedness causes mood change and character change to saying that damage has a consistent and predictable effect on personality, such as raising E or N for instance. Since mood and character changes can go in many directions, it may be fairer to conclude that damagedness is related to a 'breakdown' of personality, i.e. the patient's habits, preferences, coping processes, regulatory functions, self-concept and so on, that have been built up over the years, suffer some kind of non-specific blow.

A study by Lishman (1968) on the psychiatric sequelae of head injury tends to support this view. Lishman investigated the effects of penetration head wounds in 670 cases, placing each into one of three psychiatric categories: (a) no psychiatric disability — $n = 93$, (b) mild psychiatric disability — $n = 433$, (c) severe psychiatric disability — 144. Lishman defined psychiatric disability quite widely so

Table 5.1
The percentage of cases with and without papilloedema (P+ and P—) that show mental disorders (from Hécaen, 1964)

	Presence of papilloedema		Confused states and deterioration		Disturbances of mood and character	
Site of tumour	P+ (*n*)	P— (*n*)	P+	P—	P+	P—
Frontal	60	20	63.3%	60.0%	33.3%	50.0%
Temporal	58	41	50.0%	31.7%	20.6%	24.3%
Other cortical	61	53	36.1%	26.4%	21.3%	11.3%
Mesodiencephalic	26	35	30.7%	22.8%	38.4%	8.5%
Subtentorial	57	28	28.1%	10.7%	14.0%	7.1%
Total	262	177				

Table 5.2
Relation between measures of damagedness and psychiatric disability (from Lishman, 1968)

	N	Psychiatric disability nil	mild	severe
Depth of penetration				
(a) < 3 cm	219	25%	65%	10%
(b) > 3 cm	373	9%	66%	25%
(c) To ventricles	78	6%	59%	35%
Total brain tissue destroyed				
(a) Grade 1	52	54%	33%	13%
(b) Grade 2	224	26%	35%	39%
(c) Grade 3	66	10%	17%	73%
(d) Grade 4	3	—	33%	67%
Post-traumatic amnesia				
(a) < 1 hour	329	19%	69%	12%
(b) < 7 days	131	13%	63%	24%
(c) > 7 days	210	7%	59%	34%

as to include affective, behaviour, social, somatic, obsessional and psychotic changes, for example. Such a mixed definition accords reasonably with our equally vague notion of a 'breakdown' in personality or personal functioning.

The relationship between disability and damagedness is given in Table 5.2, where it can be seen that depth of penetration, amount of tissue destroyed, and length of post-traumatic amnesia, all correlate with psychiatric disability. This relationship is *not* mediated by pure intellectual loss (which Lishman also measured) since, for example, the correlation between depth of penetration and disability ($r = .26, p < .01$) remains significant even when intellectual impairment is partialled out ($r\ 12.3 = .20, p < 01$). As a further index of damagedness, Lishman considered for each patient the number of lobes affected (maximum of four: frontal, temporal, parietal, occipital). He computed for each of the three disability categories the average number of lobes affected per patient. This figure was 1.31, 1.40 and 1.64 for the nil, mild and severe categories respectively, showing that there is a greater chance of being severely psychiatrically disabled if more lobes are damaged.

We have to conclude, therefore, that crude, global measures of brain damage most probably do relate to personality, but not in any manner that coherently relates to any particular personality theory. The relationship is, rather, a negative and destructive one, in that changes in whatever direction are likely to be detrimental to the personal functioning of the patient. At the theoretical level we might observe that integrity of personality seems to require integrity of brain.

Epilepsy and personality

The subject of epilepsy deserves a special mention separate to the discussion of damagedness even though the two are obviously related. This is because of the idiosyncratic circumstances surrounding epilepsy. Two things are particularly important. First, epilepsy, unlike the tumours and penetration aetiologies considered above, most often starts early in childhood, giving the brain time to accommodate, adapt and circumvent the problem. Second, there are the non-specific social and interpersonal factors that act on the child because of people's distrust and fear of fits themselves and epileptics in general.

It is difficult, therefore, to decide whether the often mentioned 'problem' behaviour of epileptic children is due to the direct effect of fitting itself, i.e. a direct organic assault upon behavioural self-control, or due to a reaction by the child to a stressful environment. A study by Hackney and Taylor (1976) suggests that at least the direct organic factor is relevant. Here, 30 epileptic children were matched by age, sex and IQ to 30 psychiatric cases, all 60 children having been in-patients and therefore sharing a similar environment. In a second sample a further 30 epileptics and 30 control (normal) cases were matched, but this time the epileptics were out-patients. The 120 children each had Rutter's teacher's questionnaire (B2) completed on them. On this, antisocial and neurotic items are scored 0, 1 or 2 depending on the severity of the symptom. If a child scores 9 or more then he is placed in an antisocial disorder or neurotic disorder category depending on the particular items endorsed. The results are given in Table 5.3.

That the direct brain effect of epilepsy is important is suggested by the finding that the hospital group, who had more severe epilepsy, in whom fitting was difficult to control medically, score as far more disturbed than the out-patient group. In fact the severe epileptics score as highly as the purely psychiatric group.

This very high rate of disturbance in epileptic children has been shown elsewhere. Graham and Rutter (1968, Rutter, 1977) compared disorders involving the brain with physical disorders not involving the brain, to find that prevalence of psychiatric disorder was three times higher in the brain group; see Table 5.4.

To return to the problem of social stigma and the adverse social reaction that might produce the deviant behaviour in epileptics, this may, in fact, be overstated as a factor. Seidel, Chadwick and Rutter (1975) controlled for the factor of visibility (and hence, presumably, stigma) by comparing epileptic children with those having other visible disorders such as muscular dystrophy, polio or spina bifida. Disturbance rate was still twice as high in the epileptic, brain-lesioned group, as shown in Table 5.5.

In a review of the literature in this area, Rutter (1977) concludes that 'the beha-

Table 5.3
Scores of epileptics, normals and psychiatric children on teacher's rating scale (from Hackney and Taylor, 1976)

	In hospital		Out of hospital	
	Epileptics	Psychiatric controls	Epileptics	Normal controls
Mean score	10.8	11.4	4.9	2.8*
Mean no. items	8.5	8.3	4.4	2.3†
No. $\geq$ 9	17	18	5	3
Antisocial	8	7	1	1
Neurotic	9	11	4	2‡
Score 0-4	6	8	13	24‡
5-8	7	4	12	3‡
9-16	10	9	5	3‡
17+	7	9	0	0‡

* p. diff .05
† p. diff .01
‡ p. $<$ .01 on x^2

Table 5.4
Prevalence of psychiatric disorder in neuro-epileptic children aged 5-14 years attending school (reproduced from Graham and Rutter, 1968)

	With psychiatric disorder (No.)	(%)	Total
General population (10- and 11-year old children)	144	6.6	2189
Physical disorders not involving brain	16	11.5	139
Blind only	1	16.6	6
Deaf only	2	15.4	13
Lesion at or below brain stem	2	13.3	15
Miscellaneous physical disorders	11	10.3	107
Brain disorder	34	34.3	99
Uncomplicated epilepsy	18	28.6	63
Lesion above brain stem (no fits)	9	37.5	24
Lesion above brain stem (with fits)	7	58.3	12

Table 5.5
Prevalence of psychiatric disorder in brain-lesioned (epileptic) children and in children with visible peripheral damage

	Brain lesion (n = 33)	Peripheral (n = 42)
Deviant score on teacher's scale	30%	10%
Deviant score on parental scale	25%	13%
Disturbed at interview	45%	29%
Psychiatrically rated as disturbed	24%	12%

vioural stereotype of the brain damaged child must be firmly rejected'. In other words, epilepsy may have a marked effect on personal functioning but is not a stereotyped and predictable one. The same holds true for adult epileptics for whom there is no real epileptic 'type'. Admittedly, Richards (1952) did publish an epilepsy scale based on the MMPI, but these personality findings have perpetually been found non-replicable (see Rosenman and Lucik, 1970).

It seems that we can consider epilepsy as just another index of damagedness that has detrimental effects on personal and social functioning in non-specific directions. Indeed, Lishman (1968) found in his study that the onset of fits had exactly the same relationship to severity of psychiatric disorder as did other parameters of degree of damagedness such as depth of penetration and number of lobes affected. The evidence accrued from epileptic studies is, then, roughly congruent with the notion that brain and personality integrity are related.

Lateralisation of brain damage and personality

Having dealt with the global concept of damagedness, we can begin to consider the question of more precise localisation of lesions. The left v. right distinction seems a reasonable place to start since the left and right sides of both brain and body have long historical connections with different facets of human experience, life and personality. As shown in Table 5.6, Ornstein (1972) groups together characteristics of 'the left' and 'the right', to form an intuitively (right-brained) coherent picture of the two. Here, there are two basic hypotheses to investigate: (a) that the two hemispheres give rise to sequelae of differing severity, (b) that lesions to the left and right brain give rise to different kinds of personality dysfunction.

Flor-Henry (1969, 1973) found strong evidence that lesions to the left hemisphere have a more severe effect on functioning. He studied a group of 50 patients who were diagnosed as both psychotic and epileptic. Compared to a control group of non-psychotic, matched epileptics, they contained a much higher proportion of left lesions, as shown in Table 5.7 in which only cases of unilateral damage are considered.

The finding that left lesions are more associated with a severe illness is echoed in Lishman's study in which he takes the unilaterally lesioned cases within the nil, mild and severe psychiatric disability groups, and looks at the ratio of left to right cases (Table 5.8). With increasing severity there is a greater proportion of left lesions, although the result fails to reach statistical significance ($\chi^2 = 1.82$). However, when Lishman considered only temporal lesions, the marked left-right differences found by Flor-Henry were more clearly replicated. Since Flor-Henry's cases were all temporal epileptics, this might have been expected, and demonstrates something of an interaction between lobe effects and laterality effects. However, lobe and laterality main effects and lobe x laterality interactions are not necessarily easily replicable.

In this respect, Shaffer, Chadwick and Rutter (1975) gave the teacher's rating scale described earlier to 98 children who had suffered visible damage to the cortex after compound depressed fractures. Although the children, as a group, showed very elevated scores in agreement with the damagedness hypothesis, left lesions did not have a greater impact on psychiatric disorder than did right lesions. Nor was there any lobe effect or lobe x laterality interaction, as indicated in Table 5.9.

Table 5.6
Two modes of consciousness: a tentative dichotomy (from Ornstein, 1972)

Source		
Many sources	Day	Night
Blackburn	Intellectual	Sensuous
Oppenheimer	Time, history	Eternity, timelessness
Deikman	Active	Receptive
Polanyi	Explicit	Tacit
Levy, Sperry	Analytic	Gestalt
Domhoff	Right body	Left body
Many sources	Left hemisphere	Right hemisphere
Bogen	Propositional	Appositional
Lee	Lineal	Nonlineal
Luria	Sequential	Simultaneous
Semmes	Focal	Diffuse
I Ching	The creative: heaven	The receptive: earth
	Masculine, Yang	Feminine, Yin
I Ching	Light	Dark
I Ching	Time	Space
Many sources	Verbal	Spatial
Many sources	Intellectual	Intuitive
Jung	Causal	Acausal
Vedanta	Buddhi	Manas
Bacon	Argument	Experience

Table 5.7
Laterality of epilepsy (unilateral foci) (from Flor-Henry, 1969)

	Psychotics	Controls
Right	9	25
Left	19	13

$x^2 = 7.3, p < .01$

Given Lishman's non-significant trend and Shaffer et al.'s no trend at all, we have to conclude that the laterality effect may not be a strong parameter with regard to severity.

Turning to the nature of the disorder, rather than its simple severity, both Lishman's and Flor-Henry's studies suggest that different types of psychiatric disablement ensue from left as opposed to right lesioning. In Lishman's case the effects of left damage were primarily intellectual (IQ, dysphasia and memory) whereas right lesions led to more personality-related problems (depression, irritability, apathy, facile or childish behaviours, somatic complaints, 'frontal lobe syndrome', and 'post-traumatic syndrome'). Flor-Henry's relevant findings are given in Table 5.10. It can be seen that right lesions are especially represented in manic depressive states, reflecting somewhat the emotional or mood disturbances of Lishman's right cases.

One further piece of evidence that left and right lesions cause differing personality problems comes from research with the Minnesota Multiphasic Personality Inventory (MMPI see Table 5.11 for a list of scales). Louks et al. (1976) matched 15 left *S*s to 15 right cases (using the Reitan-Halstead battery for lateralisation) and administered the neurotic and psychotic scales from the MMPI, to yield a P-N index of L + Pa + Sc — Hy — Pt. The results, in Table 5.12, show that

Table 5.8
Laterality of lesion and psychiatric disability (from Lishman, 1977)

	Psychiatric disability		
	nil	mild	severe
No. with unilateral lesions	71	92	108
% having left lesion	51%	56%	62%
% having right lesion	49%	44%	38%

Table 5.9
Mean scores on teacher's questionnaire

	Laterality	
	left	right
Lobe, frontal	8.23	8.22
temporal	6.37	6.57
parieto-occipital	10.00	7.50

Laterality, lobe and laterality x lobe effects are NS
on two-way ANOVA

left cases are higher on psychotic features of the MMPI giving schizoid and paranoid responses, for example, while right cases show more neurotic features, responding in a more hysterical, introverted and fearful manner.

There is, then, a rough and ready alignment between Lishman's, Flor-Henry's and Louks' findings — one might say that left lesions give rise to cognitive and thought disturbances, whereas right lesions lead to affective and emotional problems. There are at least two possible reasons for the obtained differences although in neither case are the mechanisms clear: (a) language is in the left hemisphere so that its disruption may lead to changes in the verbal control of behaviour and thinking, a consideration which will be taken up later when aphasia and the left temporal lobe are discussed in detail, (b) functions in the left are more tightly arranged into centres or cortical nuclei while the right arrangements of function are more diffuse (Semmes, 1972) so that left lesions are more likely to cause specific cognitive defects whereas right lesions disturb functions that require diffuse cortical representation such as spatial awareness, and, possibly, emotional or affective analysis.

As a final point in this discussion, it should be remembered that bilateral lesions are probably more disruptive than unilateral ones, in line with the dam-

Table 5.10
Laterality and type of psychosis (Flor-Henry, 1969)

	Manic depressive	Mixed	Confusional	Schizophrenic
Right	44%	18%	11%	9.5%
Left	22%	36%	44.5%	43%
Bilateral	33%	46%	44.5%	47.5%

$x^2 = 4.4; p$ .05

Table 5.11
Minnesota multiphasic personality inventory: scale names, abbreviations and a guide to their meaning

?	Question	No. of items in 'cannot say' category
L	Lie	Social desirability of responses
F	Validity	A judgement of test validity (not a scale)
K	K	Correction factor
Hs	Hypochondriasis	Concern with bodily functions
D	Depression	Neurotic depression
Hy	Hysteria	Conversion-hysteria type symptoms
Pd	Psychopathic deviate	Absence of emotional response
Mf	Masculinity-femininity	Gender identity of interests
Pa	Paranoia	Suspiciousness and over-sensitivity
Pt	Psychaesthenia	Phobias and compulsive behaviour
Sc	Schizophrenia	Bizarre, unusual thoughts and behaviour
Ma	Hypomania	Over-productivity in thought and action

agedness hypothesis. For example, Rutter (1977, Rutter et al. 1970) notes that in children psychiatric disorder is significantly more common with bilateral than unilateral lesions, and in Flor-Henry's data the bilateral:unilateral ratio is his psychotic group was 1:1.27 whereas it was 1:3.45 in his control subjects. In the last study to be mentioned, Meier and French (1965) administered the MMPI to 53 cases of psychomotor epilepsy. They plotted MMPI profiles separately for bilateral and unilateral groups as shown in Fig. 5.1, finding that bilateral scores are very distinctly elevated on most of the scales. Again we see that the more brain that is damaged, the more personality is detrimentally affected.

An important suggestion can now be made in regard to brain-personality relationships. It is that given the indication of left-right differences, an organic

Table 5.12
Personality disturbances in left and right lesion cases (from Louks et al., 1976)

	Left		Right		t
	X	σx	X	σx	
Age	46.9	9.2	45.3	11.3	0.4, NS
Average impairment rating	2.4	0.62	2.1	1.0	—0.28, NS
P-N index	61.5	26.1	38.1	32.7	2.17, $p<.05$

theory of personality cannot be based solely on general properties of the brain. This may seem an obvious point, but inhibition-excitation models and the theories of strength, mobility and so on tend to ignore the different structure and functions of the various systems in which the general properties might be measured. Therefore, in order to predict more accurately the effects of raised inhibition or increased strength, we need to know whether the changes occur, say, in the left or right brain, or in which lobe, or in the anterior or posterior regions. This will become more evident as various lobes and systems within the brain are considered.

Fig. 5.1 Mean MMPI profiles of the bilateral and unilateral EEG abnormality group, (from Meier and French, 1965)

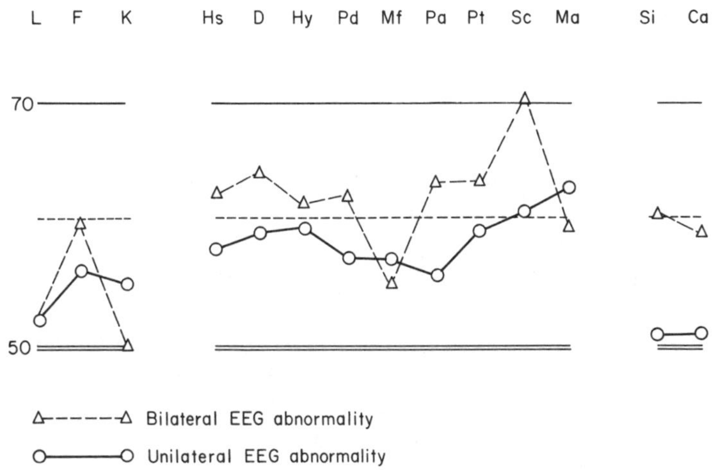

6 The role of specific lobes for personality

Having dealt with indices of more generalised damage we shall now consider findings that relate to more circumscribed areas of brain, especially those that concern psychosurgery. The surprising thing here is that, although the details of brain connections have been mapped in a voluminous literature, the theoretical models that psychosurgeons employ appear extremely simple. For example, the crude model depicted in Fig. 6.1 has been seriously put forward as a summary of psychosurgical premises by Obrador (1972). In stark contrast to the lack of theory as to *why* a particular area of brain should be destroyed there are very lengthy descriptions as to *how* to go about it.

The frontal lobes

First, a brief neural description of the frontal lobes, based on reviews by Nauta (1971) and Homskaya (1973). Afferents are received from the visual, auditory and somatic sensory areas (corticocortical or associative links); from the olfactory system; and from the thalamus, septal and related limbic regions. Efferents are sent to the anterior temporal cortex; to the inferior parietal lobule; to the cingulate and parahippocampal gyri (all cortical projections); and to the limbic system, especially the hypothalamus (subcortical projections). The frontal lobes in man are not homogenous with regard to function, so that separate attributes are often assigned to various regions. Writers differ over the details of this heterogeneity, but all distinguish between the prefrontal cortex and the more posterior

Fig. 6.1 'Preferential' areas, for surgical intervention (from Obrador, 1972)

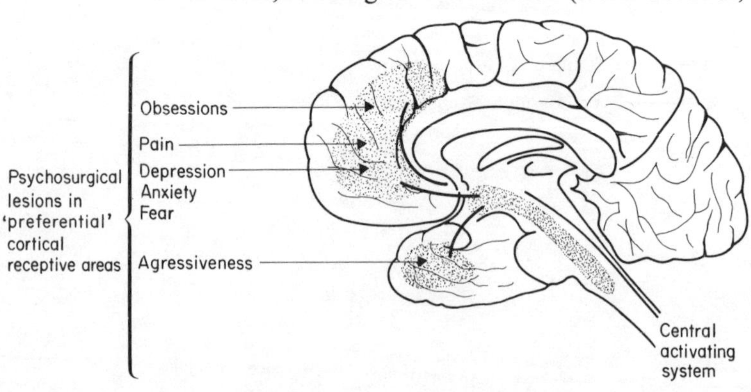

motor regions and most would see the orbital region as being especially linked to the limbic system. Heterogeneity can also be deduced by considering the symptoms attached to particular lesions. For example, Le Beau (1954) claims to distinguish five 'frontal syndromes' centred upon lesions in (a) the dorsal convexity, (b) the rostral convexity, (c) the frontal pole (d) the orbital region, and (e) the cingulate gyrus. Others (e.g. Meyer and Beck, 1954) accent the equipotentiality of the different prefrontal regions and emphasise the sheer quantity of tissue destroyed.

Obviously, the possibility of heterogeneity makes the results of different studies harder to compare, and the search for 'the' frontal syndrome difficult. At the very least we need to discriminate between those surgical procedures that attack the brain from above (as in the standard leucotomy) and those that attack from below (orbital undercutting), given the latter's special association with the limbic system and the brain stem.

No large scale review of the frontal lobes will be attempted here since so many others exist (see Willett, 1960; Blakemore, 1967; and Passingham, 1970). Just two hypotheses will be considered: (a) that frontal lesions increase extraversion as predicted by Eysenk and Gray, (b) that in accord with the damagedness concept, frontal lesions will produce detrimental personality changes.

Studies that report standardised personality tests are few and far between, but a few exist, originating with the use of the MMPI. One of the first such studies, and also one of the worst, was by Anderson and Harvik (1950), who conclude 'the mean personality type of the frontal group to be capable of description somewhat as follows: accepting, non-irritable, non anxious, affable, easy-going, and possessed of a relatively low general level of aspiration'. This sounds like an increase in extraversion and a beneficial lowering of neuroticism, but this is a sweeping conclusion for a study on only 16 frontals badly matched to 27 parietal lesions. Frontals were higher on *K*, and parietals higher on *F*, D, Pt and Ie (see Fig. 6.2 and refer to table 5.11 for a list of MMP 1 scales). Since there was no knowledge of pre-scores and no comparison with any normal matched controls, very little sense can actually be made of the frontal's profiles. However, when pre-scores *are* known, two of the above scales, D and Pt, seem to be relevant, for scores on them significantly fell in 21 prefrontal leucotomy cases tested before and after their operations by Vidor (1951). In a similar and more recent study by Walsh (1977) 100 modified leucotomy cases were tested on the MMPI before and after their operation. Once again scores on these two scales reflecting depressive and anxiety symptoms (D and Pt) changed markedly for the better ($p < .001$ in both instances). This was part of an overall pattern of beneficial change in that scores on Hy, Pa and Sc also fell significantly.

Encouraged by these and other studies, Friedman (1950) tried to develop a parietal-frontal scale, finding in his own study that parietals were higher on *F*, Hs, D, Hy, Pt, Sc and Si, and lower on *K* than frontals. Once again, the scales D and Pt figure in the results. However, the eventual scale suffered considerably

Fig. 6.2 The mean *t* score profiles for 16 cases of frontal lobe brain damage and 27 cases of brain damage involving the parietal lobe (from Andersen and Harvik, 1950)

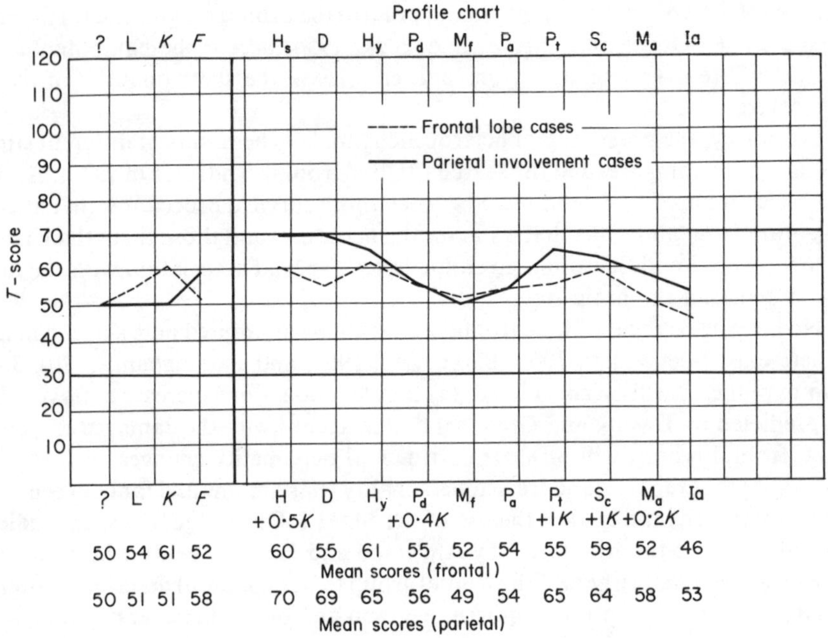

from regression to the mean effects when attempts were made to replicate it (Williams, 1952; Meier, 1969).

An attempt to construct a similar scale, called the caudal scale to measure the caudality-rostrality of lesioning, was reported by Williams (1952). Using 48 frontals, 48 parietals and 20 temporals he reports some difficulty in differentiating between the groups — especially between the frontals and temporals. The final scale consisted of 33 items, many of which are interesting, since in a way they tell us more about frontals than knowing their scores on complex scales such as Ie or Ip or P-N. Here are some of the pertinent items, together with the direction in which frontals score:

I enjoy the excitement of a good crowd	true
I am a good mixer	true
I find it hard to make talk when I meet new people	false
I practically never blush	true
I usually have to stop and think before I act even in trifling matters	false
I am usually calm and not easily upset	true

I brood a great deal	false
Most of the time I feel blue	false
At times I feel like smashing things	false

These items suggest a positive change in both social behaviour and mood, which, when coupled with the previous hint of change in D (depression) and Pt (anxiety and absessional symptoms), can be taken as indicating raised E and lowered N.

Looking for more definite evidence relating to extraversion, we might consider the study of Post et al. (1968) who examine the changes in interpersonal behaviour shown by 64 modified leucotomy cases (for the treatment of depression, pain and obsessions). It is a strange study, in that the basic data were in the form of written précis of the patient's functioning at various times before and after the operation, these précis being made up by a social worker who interviewed the patients and examined the case notes. Functioning in several areas (including those that we are interested in here — 'close personal relationships' and 'distant personal relationships') was then assessed by blind ratings of the précis by psychiatrists. It seems pointless having blind ratings when the original data (i.e. the précis) were not collected or extracted blind. Bearing this possible bias in mind, the results have been displayed in Table 6.1.

As can be seen from the means in the table, improvement in interpersonal functioning was slight and non-significant. In a detailed analysis of results, Post shows how two-thirds of the patients suffered undesirable leucotomy effects. In the case of personality changes, these were characterised as mild outspokenness; being a little slipshod; anergic, or slow; showing slight lack of feeling; emotional lability.

It is apparent, then, that a study which, despite its methodological faults, could well have picked up changes in an extraverted direction, failed to do so.

Table 6.1
The number of frontal patients scoring at each rating level

	Intimate relations			Distant relations		
Score	pre-	1 year	3 year	pre-	1 year	3 year
Very poor 1	0	0	0	1	0	1
2	3	0	1	4	2	3
3	10	3	7	9	4	5
4	18	20	12	20	14	11
5	12	17	19	13	15	17
Normal 6	8	11	12	2	14	12
Mean	4.23	4.71	4.67	3.78	4.53	4.37

Turning to a specific aspect of extraversion, it is often cited that frontal cases become sexually more liberal, in line with the fact that extraverts have higher libido and enjoy more frequent and varied sex. This is not the case. Post did not find it; nor did Miller (1954) in 147 standard lobotomy case; nor did Pippard (1955) in 114 cases of rostral leucotomy; nor did Freeman (1973) who cites that fact that of 64 patients given the Kinsey sexual interview before and after topectomy, 10 took more interest in sex and 10 took less interest.

Personality changes that do accrue from frontal lesions are in fact more as described by Post. Pippard (1955) too describes less drive, less enthusiasm, less of a go-getter, things are more of an effort, less concern for others, selfish, diminished regard for appearance, irritability; and Miller (1954) describes similar changes in a passive, resistive and negativistic direction.

The lack of relationship between extraversion and frontal lesions is emphasised by two studies that used an actual questionnaire measure of the trait. In the first study, Levinson and Meyer (1965) gave the Mandsley Personality Inventory (MPI) to 179 frontals to find that their mean E-score of 24.34 was not above the published norm of 24.91. A further 29 cases had both pre- and post-tests on the MPI and here there was a trend for E-scores to rise (16.31 to 18.23) but it was not significant. In the second study, Kelly et al. (1966) gave the MPI to 40 modified leucotomy cases both before and after the operation. The trend for a rise in E (15.4 to 17.2) was not significant.

One more line of evidence linking frontal functioning with extraversion should be considered, for it has often been pointed out that frontals score like extraverts on laboratory tests. However, it is more parsimonious simply to say that frontal lesions cause a performance decrement. In two major studies by Tow (1955) and Petrie (1952) we see that: full scale IQ goes down; verbal IQ and vocabulary go down; matrices IQ goes down; Porteus maze IQ goes down; word fluency down; word similarity down; object sorting down; persistence down; accuracy on letter cancellation and tracing down. The only change that might be described as positive is an increase in speed. But it is not a controlled, useful increase in speed, more a failure to undertake the task responsibly — 'slapdash work' as Tow describes it.

If the frontal lobes are the seat of extraversion, the evidence is unimpressive. However, the matter cannot be considered entirely closed as in a recent report by Smith, Kiloh and Boots (1977) it is suggested that 30 months after prefrontal leucotomy, extraversion scores *are* above the pre-operative level (6.5 *v* 10.3, $p < .005$, $n = 31$). This was seen within the context of a quite considerable beneficial change in mood state since scores on the Hamilton anxiety scale, the Hamilton depression scale, the Beck depression scale and the Neuroticism scale, also reduced significantly (mainly at the .001 level). Therefore the field is not without some conflicting data, but this study by Smith et al. would seem to be an exception to the general findings regarding frontal lesioning and extraversion. It could be that Smith's group was so terribly introverted in the first place (mean of

6.5) that some regression to the mean was only to be expected (i.e. part or all of the shift in E scores could be a statistical artifact).

There are two general findings that stand up across most of the studies, however. First, the postoperative prevalence of reduced behavioural activity variously described as apathy, inertia and the like (Post et al., 1968; Miller, 1954; Pippard, 1955; Tan et al., 1971; Freeman, 1973) which may be accounted for by a change in cortical arousal induced by disturbing frontal-brain-stem connections and evidenced by increased α-wave activity in the EEG, as found by Homskaya (1973) and Miller (1954), whose results are depicted in Fig. 6.3. Second, a reduction in unpleasant moods variously described as depression, anxiety and neurotic fear (Anderson and Harvik, 1950; Friedman, 1950; Williams, 1952; Marks et al., 1966; Post et al., 1968; Tan et al., 1971). Whether one sees this second effect as beneficial or not depends on semantics, for they could be rewritten with a different flavour: irresponsible attitude to problems; lack of awareness of problems; blunting of effect; reduced insight into personal predicaments; inappropriate emotions.

Perhaps one could say that in a normal individual, frontal lesions will be seen as having a detrimental effect on personality, in accordance with the damagedness hypothesis (e.g. Table 6.2), whereas in the severely disabled population who

Fig. 6.3. Graphic representation showing the increase in alpha incidence after lobotomy. A fairly even distribution of cases in the 20 to 80 per cent range is apparent before the operation, whereas the same population 4 to 6 weeks after operation shows a shift towards a higher alpha incidence, with a concentration of cases in the 60 to 80 per cent range (EEG body; from Miller, 1954)

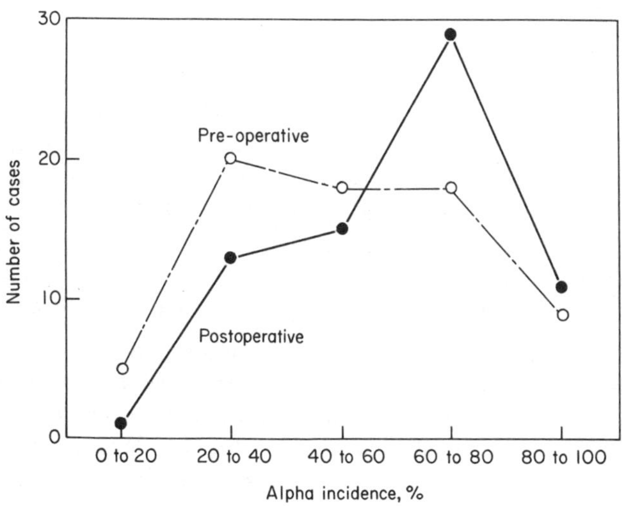

Table 6.2
Disturbances of mood and character in frontal tumour cases (from Hécaen, 1964)

	Series			
	I	II	Total	Percentage
Total no. of cases	80	51	131	
Total cases with disturbances of mood and character	30	21	51	38.9
Specific symptoms				
Irritability	13	8	21	16.0
Euphoria	17	9	26	19.8
Agressivity	2	1	3	2.3
Depression	6	8	14	10.7
mild	4	5	9	5.9
severe	2	3	5	3.8
Emotional instability	4	1	5	3.8
Mood swings	5	4	9	6.1
Anxiety	0	2	2	1.5
Bulimia	1	0	1	0.7
Hypersexuality	1	0	1	0.7
Psychosis	3	3	6	4.6

undergo deliberate surgical lesioning, these detrimental effects are milder than the original symptoms and directly inhibit such symptoms (e.g. Table 6.3). The mechanism mediating these mood changes is likely to be the severing of fronto-limbic connections. For this reason we shall consider next, lesions specifically to these limbic system connections that provide access to all kinds of 'pleasure' and 'unpleasure' centres (Weil, 1974).

Amygdalectomy

The role of the limbic system (Fig. 6.4) in emotion, motivation, drive and so forth has been well documented elsewhere and will not be repeated here (see Maclean and Delgado, 1953; Ursin, 1960; Isaccson 1974; Weil, 1974). We are mainly interested in just a few of the limbic connections that have come to be known as Papez's circuit, after the theory of emotion proposed by Papez (1937). The crux of the mechanism can be described succinctly as follows

> The central emotive process of cortical origin may then be conceived as being built up in the hippocampal formation and as being transferred to the mamillary body and thence through the anterior thalamic nuclei to the cortex of the gyrus cinguli. The cortex of the cingular gyrus may be looked on as the receptive region for the experiencing of emotion as the result of

Table 6.3
Symptoms altered by orbital undercutting (Hetherington et al., 1972)

Symptom	Worse	No change	Improved	Total
Anxiety	0	1	13	14
Depression	0	1	13	14
Phobias	0	0	6	6
Compulsions	1	1	9	11
Hypochondriasis	1	0	6	7
Insomnia	1	2	8	11
Care of property	1	1	4	6
Concentration	2	0	9	11
Volubility	2	1	7	10
Insight	2	1	6	9
Self-confidence	3	1	10	14
Interest in life	4	0	10	14
Affect	3	0	3	6
Personal habits	3	0	4	7
Initiative	5	0	7	12
Memory	6	1	4	11
Outspokenness	6	1	3	10
Hostility	6	1	4	11

> impulses coming from the hypothalamic region, in the same way as the area striata is considered the receptive cortex for photic excitations coming from the retina. . . . This circuit would explain how emotion may arise in two ways: as a result of psychic activity and as a consequence of hypothalamic activity. (Papez, 1937)

If the picture is filled in with a few other relevant connections, particularly the basolateral loop, the model can be described schematically as in Fig. 6.5.

It can be seen that the effect this 'emotional' circuit has on cortical processing could be disrupted by appropriate lesions, particularly if placed in (a) the lower medial quadrant of the frontal lobes, (b) the postorbital gyrus or its projections, (c) the cingulate gyrus, or (d) the amygdala. In each case, frontal-limbic connections would be disturbed. The probable effect of such lesions would be to inhibit emotionally instigated behaviours. In this respect, Kelly (1973) notes that animals become less fearful and aggressive after cingulate lesions; Vaernet and Madsen (1970) point out that patients feel fear and apprehension if the amygdala is electrically stimulated during temporal lobe operations; and Narabayashi et al. (1963) remind us that after operations on the deep structures of the temporal lobe (i.e. amygdala and hippocampus) to remove epilepsy, the consequent changes in behaviour, notably beneficial changes in temper tantrums and aggressive episodes, are often more pronounced than any reduction in fit frequency.

Drawing from such evidence, Narabayashi et al. (1963) undertook a series of

Fig. 6.4 Schema of the limbic system. OB olfactory bulb, LOT lateral olfactory striae, INS insula, UB uncinate bundle, DB diagonal band of Broca, AMYG amygdala, SCR subcallosal radiations, HYP hypothalamus, AT anterior thalamus, MB mammillary body, MTT mammillothalamic trace (Vicq D'Azyr's tracts), ATR anterior thalamic radiations, ST stria terminalis, HAB habenula, MFB medial forebrain bundle, SM stria medullaris, HPT habenulointerpeducunlar tract (fasciculus retroflexus of Meynert), IP interpeduncular nucleus, LMA limbic midbrain area of Nauta, G nucleus of Gudden, CG central gray, CCF corpus callosum (from Ballantine et al., 1967)

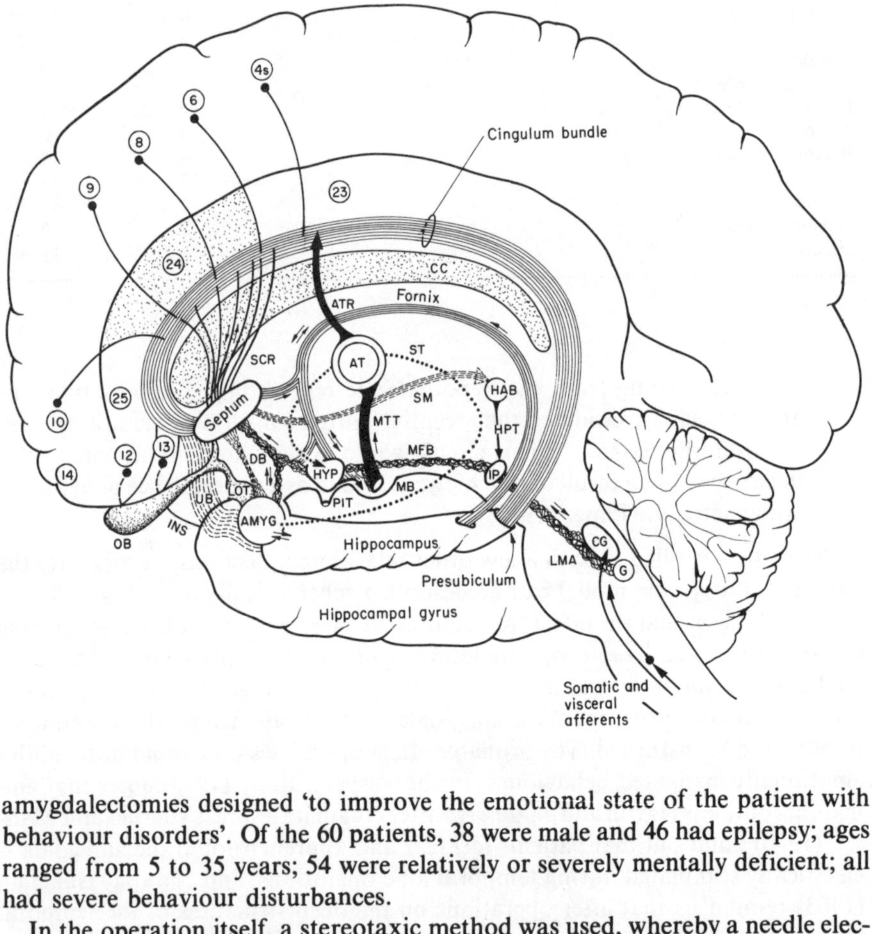

amygdalectomies designed 'to improve the emotional state of the patient with behaviour disorders'. Of the 60 patients, 38 were male and 46 had epilepsy; ages ranged from 5 to 35 years; 54 were relatively or severely mentally deficient; all had severe behaviour disturbances.

In the operation itself, a stereotaxic method was used, whereby a needle electrode is passed through a burr hole in the frontoparietal region into the amygdaloid nucleus, visualisation of the electrode placement being achieved by concurrent air encephalography. Electrophysiological data, continuously collected via the electrode, also assisted accurate placement. The eventual destruction of the nucleus was achieved by the injection of oil, wax and lipiodal, producing a lesion of 8 to 10 mm in diameter. The injected material is not absorbed but is semipermanent and can be measured by X-ray.

Despite the surgeon's claims of 'careful examination and testing of all patients' and 'careful and repeated observations', the outcome measure was crude, being a four-point rating scale: A greatly improved, becoming calm, obedient and social adaptation being possible; B moderately improved, easier to control, calm and with better concentration; C slightly improved, excitation reduced; D no change. The numbers within each category after up to four years' follow-up were 29, 22, 7 and 2 respectively, i.e. a claimed success rate of 85 per cent. The success of the operation seems to depend partly on the exact site of lesioning within the amygdala, since 72 per cent of lesions to the medial nucleus produced a grade A result compared with only 9 per cent when the lateral nucleus was lesioned (Narabayashi and Shima, 1973).

As a scientific inquiry, the Narabayaski study leaves so much to be desired that it is difficult to evaluate the effects of amygdala lesions in humans. In particular, we have no detailed description of behavioural changes, because of the apparent complete lack of standardised data collection. The rating scale that we are offered is next to useless since it lumps together many different aspects of behaviour including concentration, school performance, cognitive abilities, aggression, emotionality, social integration, hyperactivity and so on. However, the terms that are used most frequently centre on calmness, obedience, controllability and lack of emotional outbursts.

Fig. 6.5 Diagrammatic representation of Papez's circuit

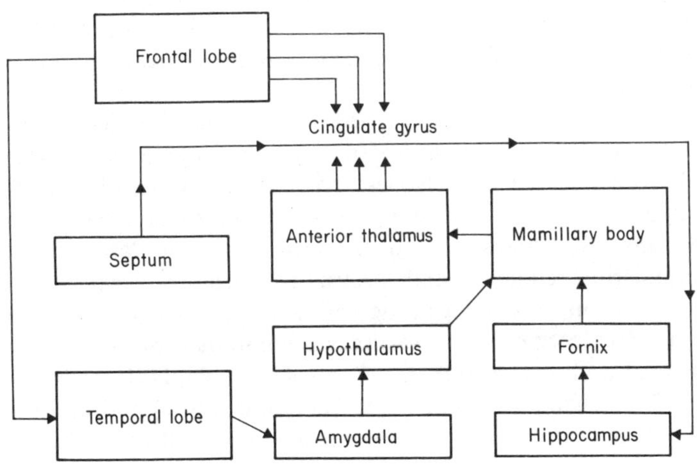

Assuming that the rating scale *mainly* reflects the flavour of these factors, the figure of 85 per cent is high enough to suggest that even taking into account rater bias and spontaneous recovery, amygdalectomy is having some kind of placating effect. Narabayashi hastens to observe that this behavioural sedation is not of the detrimental kind seen after frontal lesions

> In none of our cases, even those subjected to bilateral amygdalotomy, did we observe the passive, emotionless stage with marked inertia or severe loss of interest in the environment, which was observed so frequently after prefrontal leukotomy or dorsomedial thalamotomy. Following amygdalotomy, the patients simply acted as feebleminded or rather stupid school children.

In a second clinical trial of amygdalectomy, Vaernet and Madsen (1970) operated on 12 patients who were extremely aggressive (they were either personality disordered or chronic schizophrenic). Of these, two had had a previous cingulectomy and five a frontal lobotomy. Vaernet and Madsen again used a stereotaxic technique, bilaterally electrocoagulating the amygdala, to find 'marked improvement' in 11 of the 12 cases. Again, there is a complete absence of any reasonable measures of behavioural, cognitive and affective change. In fact, between the Narabayashi and Vaernet and Madsen studies, we have two of the worst possible examples of methodology in psychosurgery.

The use of amygdalectomy as a means of inhibiting aggression has become quite a common procedure, and so we shall consider here some of the reports from various centres of neurosurgery scattered world-wide.

Mark, Sweet and Ervin (1972) treated 10 cases of uncontrolled fear, violence, or both, by unilateral or bilateral stereotaxic amygdalotomy. A slight refinement was that after the first set of lesions, the electrodes remained in place for up to a year so that further lesions could be made if no therapeutic outcome were apparent. The immediate effect on aggression was to completely relieve it in 9 cases so that only one derived no benefit. However, in only 3 of these 9 cases has the change lasted for more than one year, and 4 of the 9 cases had a recurrence of symptoms within one year.

One of the most extensive series carried out, in terms of subject numbers that in most studies tend to be small, is reported by Balasubramaniam, Ramanujam, Kanaka and Ramanurthi (1972). No less than 128 cases were subjected to amygdalotomy in a period of 6 years (of which 14 went on to have further lesions in the hypothalamus, reticular system, or temporal cortex), for 'assaultive', 'hyperkinesis', 'wandering tendency' and 'destructive' behaviour patterns. Clinical improvement was on a six-point rating scale A to F, of which the last point was 'died' and A represented complete recovery of emotional control without drugs. The numbers at each rating were A = 9, B = 45, C = 45, D (transient improvement) = 15, E (no change) - 5, and F = 9. Therefore only 29 subjects (9 of whom died) failed to gain any lasting postoperative benefit. Of the 20 living. unimproved patients, 8 were subjected to a hypothalotomy after which 6 showed some lasting beneficial change.

Once again, the absence of useful psychological measures is conspicuous, due, say Balasubramaniam et al. to the fact that 'in many others [cases] rapport could not be established between the patient and the psychologist'. This is nonsense. Direct observation measures and functional analysis techniques do not require patient co-operation at all.

A final study is well worth mentioning as it represents a real attempt to come to grips with the problem of assessment. Hitchcock et al. (1972) acknowledge that far too much attention had been given to aggression — 'in addition, seconday behaviour disturbances, apathy, stealing and other affective disturbances' were also part of the picture. Therefore, they constructed for use in their department (at the Royal Infirmary, Edinburgh) the cognitive and personality test battery given in Fig. 6.6. They make the extremely valid point that one needs a *special* assessment approach for psychosurgical operations — 'routine psychological assessments were found to be quite inadequate and a more extensive assessment procedure was devised with particular emphasis on observational techniques, self-ratings, and methods yielding information about the process of change over a period of time'. Hitchcock et al. are now using the test battery in a trial of bilateral stereotactic amygdalotomy, and so the eventual published results are looked forward to with interest. A preliminary report suggests that when carefully standardised measures are used in preference to simple rating scales, the effects of the operation seem far less estensive (Hitchcock et al., 1973).

Overall, we may conclude that the effects seem dramatic enough to warrant the claim that destruction of the amygdala reduces violent, aggressive and assaultive acts. But several points need to be borne in mind for future research: (a) data

Fig. 6.6 Test battery for amgdalotomy (Hitchcock et al., 1972)

Cognitive tests	*Personality and behaviour*
1 Raven's matrices	1 Cattell 16 P.F.
2 Mill Hill vocabulary	2 Multiple-affect adjective checklist
3 Porteus maze	3 Gottschalk scales
4 Graham-Kendall memory for designs	4 Personality and Personal illness questionnaire (Caine, Foulds and Hope)
5 Sentence repetition	5 Hargreaves nursing rating scale
6 Williams, new-word learning test	6 Various visual analogue scales for various continua
7 Williams, delayed recall test	

is lacking on the remission of symptoms in the longer term, (b) much of the data has been collected on mentally subnormal patients who may, therefore, constitute a population with abnormal, or already damaged brains, (c) different facets of aggression have not been delineated, in the way that aggression or toughmindedness as a trait should have been distinguished from specific behavioural assaults, (d) the claim that the operation does not produce an adverse personality type (as in the standard leucotomy) must remain only a claim until suitable multiple-baseline methodologies have been employed that deliberately set out to assess personality traits other than the primary target of aggression, (e) the effects on negative mood states such as anxiety and depression is unclear due to this lack of appropriate assessment.

Cingulectomy

The state of affairs regarding the evaluation of the cingulate operation is far better, owing to two reports by Kelly et al. (1973) and Mitchell-Heggs, Kelly and Richardson (1976).

In the first study, Kelly et al. (1973) report the progress of 40 patients six weeks after surgery. Of the 40 patients, 17 were suffering from chronic obsessions, 5 were depressed, 9 chronically and severely anxious, 6 were schizophrenic, one case was of continued depersonalisation feelings, one was anorexic and there was one personality disorder. As for the operation itself, a stereotaxic freezing technique was used, lesioning both cingulate sites and lower medial quadrant sites, as indicated in Fig. 6.7.

The overall clinical response was marked improvement in 12 cases, some improvement in 15 cases, and no change in the remaining 13 cases. More specific assessment measures showed distinct improvement in anxiety and depression across most of the patients. If we take anxiety first, the score on the neuroticism scale of the MPI fell from 30.8 to 23.1 ($p <$ 001); Taylor's manifest anxiety scale scores fell 31.9 to 24.1 ($p < .001$); scores on Hamilton's anxiety scale also fell 22.2 to 12.3 ($p < .001$); certain physiological measures of anxiety fell significantly, that is forearm blood pressure, heart rate, and systolic blood presure; and finally, an observer's rating scale of anxiety fell significantly although a self-rating scale did not. As for the depression indices, scores reduced on the Beck depression scale (26.4 to 18.7, $p < .001$) and the Hamilton depression scale (21.5 to 10.5, $p < .001$); and both observer and self-rating scales of depression exhibited significant reductions. Cognitive intellectual functions did not seem to be affected by the operation, although there was a small rise in IQ (103.9 to 106.0, $p < .05$) due mainly to a rise in performance IQ (98.3 to 102.2, $p < .01$). This change, however, would seem to be just a practice effect, which is known to be more marked on performance items. There was no change, either, in extraver-

Fig. 6.7 Lesion sites in relation to ventricles (v)

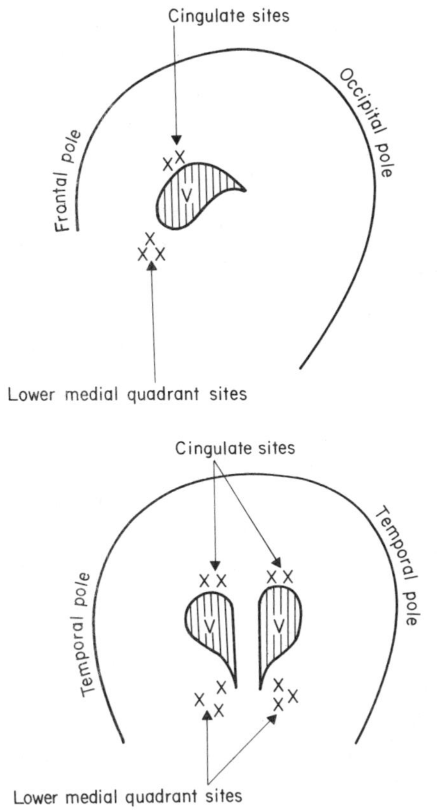

sion scores although there was a slight but non-significant rise of 12.9 to 14.2.

It is worth digressing slightly from Kelly's work to mention here that in another cingulectomy series Laitinen and Vilkki (1973) also gave the Eysenck personality questionnaire pre- and postoperatively in 18 cases. They, too, found an immediate decrease in neruoticism ($p < .05$) and no significant change in extraversion. The bilateral stereotactic target sites were rather different to the Kelly study, being in the most rostral part of the cingulum, just below and in front of the knee of the corpus callosum (the operation being known as an anterior mesoloviotomy).

These initial findings of short term change look promising as they suggest beneficial changes in distressing mood states, without side effects. The longer term operative effects have been charted by Mitchell-Heggs et al. (1976) who describe the outcome in 66 patients seen at least one year after the operation. The patients were 23 men and 43 women aged 21 to 65 years (mean of 38 years), who had had severely disabling symptoms for an average of 11 years. The bulk of the patients were suffering from obsessional neurosis (27), chronic anxiety (15), depression (9) and schizophreniz (7). The operative procedure was as described previously (i.e. lesioning in two cingulate sites and three lower medial quadrant sites) with the additional note that occasionally lesions were made in the genu of the corpus callosum.

Considering global change first of all: the improvement rate at 16 months was 89 per cent for the obsessionals, 66 per cent for the anxiety cases, 78 per cent for the depressives, and 86 per cent for the schizo-affective group. The details of the psychological improvement of patients are given in Table 6.4. It can be seen that the beneficial changes at six weeks are maintained through to 16 months. By far the greatest proportion of changes occur during the first six weeks with only minimal changes thereafter.

From these results, the findings in regard to anxiety and depression are more or less theoretically predictable, given that the limbic circuits that 'add emotional colouring to psychic processes (Papez, 1937)' are largely severed from the frontal cortex by the dual lesioning of frontal-hypothalmic connections and cingulum pathways, What is more surprising is the effect the operation has on obsessions, for the role of anxiety and emotion here is not clearly delineated bearing in mind that tranquillisers do not touch the problem. Indeed, if I had been asked what to predict regarding the effects of dissociating Papez's circuit in obsessionals, I would have hypothesised a continuation of all behaviour symptoms, but without the guilt and distress that the patient feels for performing the acts.

In examining the data in Table 6.4 it is clear that the operation is having some kind of *non-specific* action upon obsessions, since scores on the Leyton obsessional inventory fall just as much for the non-obsessional group as for the real obsessionals. One possible explanation concerns the way that the Leyton scale is heavily loaded with 'sickness' statements irrespective of the specific content of the 'sickness' or disorder; that as the patients felt a greater sense of well-being postoperatively, so they were less likely to respond affirmatively to *any* sickness statement regardless of its content. In other words, in the absence of actual behavioural observation data including frequency counts of obsessional acts, it is probably unwise to conclude that behavioural symptomatology has reduced even though the Leyton gives a positive result. The Kelly and Mitchell-Heggs groups are well aware of such problems, including, in addition, problems of comparing their results with spontaneous remission rates and with newer behaviour therapy techniques, and they hope to undertake a full clinical trial at some stage.

An earlier series of cingulotomy operations was studied by Ballantine et al. (1967, 1972), in 160 cases of either intractable pain or mental illness. Ballantine was particularly interested in the effects of the operation on 'mood disturbance', and therefore from the total group selected 66 who suffered under this general

Table 6.4
Mean psychometric values before and 6 weeks and 16 months after limbic leucotomy (N = 57) (from Mitchell-Heggs et al., 1976)

	pre-	6 weeks	16 months		*p* pre v. 16 months
MPI					
Neuroticism	33.8	24.2	23.8		.001
Extraversion	14.4	16.7	16.7		NS
Depression					
Beck	25.5	17.2	15.3		.001
Hamilton	22.6	10.6	12.8		.001
Anxiety					
Taylor	32.2	24.2	22.3		.001
Hamilton	24.0	12.6	14.4		.001
Middlesex Hospital Questionnaire					
Anxiety	11.6	9.1	8.3		.001
Phobic	7.5	6.0	5.8		.001
Obessional	11.3	9.1	8.6		.001
Somatic	7.8	5.2	4.5		.001
Depressive	9.9	7.5	6.9		.001
Hysteric	5.5	5.1	4.3		.001
Leyton obsessional inventory					
Symptoms	26.7	16.9	15.7		.001
Traits	12.1	9.6	9.0	n = 25	.01
Resistance	39.8	21.6	17.1	mixed	.001
Interference	41.6	21.6	16.0	diagnosis	.001
Symptoms	32.6	19.0	18.3		.001
Traits	12.5	9.6	9.0	n = 12	.05
Resistance	56.0	24.2	17.2	obsessionals	.001
Interference	57.7	20.9	14.1		.001

rubric (including depressives, obsessive compulsive neurotics, severe anxiety neuroses and anorexia nervosa). All of the 66 cases were available for follow-up for at least one year, and all had had the standard operation using stereotaxic lesioning to the cingulate bundle 2 to 4 cm posterior to the lip of the anterior horns of the ventricles.

On the basis of interviews and questionnaires, the cases were rated on a seven-point scale of improvement, as given in Fig. 6.8 for 40 psychiatric cases followed up for a period of three months to four years. Ballantine's group went on to give a further cingulotomy, destroying more tissue, in those cases that failed to respond to the first operation, to find evidence that therapeutic effect was

Fig. 6.8 Status of 40 psychiatric patients after cingulotomy (Ballantine et al., 1967)

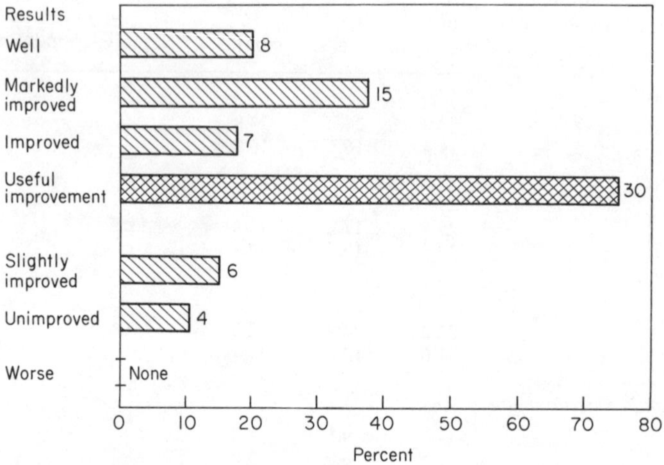

Fig. 6.9 Relationship of postoperative status to dosage after one operation and 28 repeat operations (Ballantine et al., 1972)

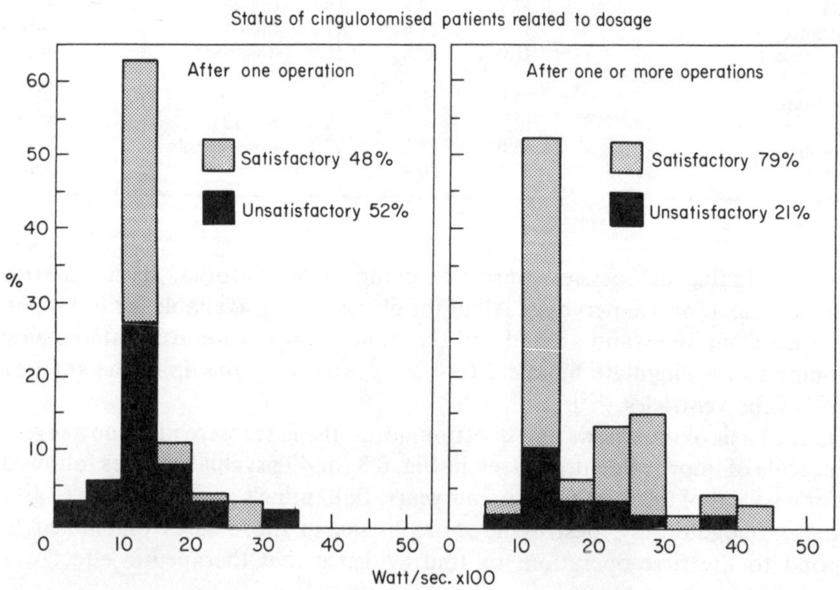

roughly in proportion to 'dosage'. The additional beneficial effects of further operations can be seen in Fig. 6.9, which indicates that outcome was satisfactory in only 48 per cent of cases after one operation, but satisfactory in 79 per cent of cases after one or more operations. Results in this figure pertain to all 66 cases, and satisfactory is defined as 'well' or 'markedly improved'. In the light of the low failure rate of 21 per cent, Ballantine et al. say that 'years should not be allowed to pass before cingulotomy is employed as an adjunct to psychiatric management'. Overall, these results are roughly in accord with the result of the Kelly group previously discussed.

Reports from three more groups will be mentioned briefly. First, Laitinen and Vilkki (1972) carried out cingulotomies on 20 patients mainly suffering from anxiety unaffected by chemotherapy. In 9 cases a good anxiolytic result was obtained, in 9 more there was a net improvement and 2 obtained no benefit. There seemed to be no cognitive deterioration, and indeed on the cases given psychometric tests, performance improved significantly on the Purdue pegboard, and on the subtests of digit span, digit symbol and block design from the WAIS. Here, it might also be mentioned that Meyer et al. (1973) similarly administered the WAIS pre- and postoperatively, this time on 30 cingulectomy cases. They, too, found a slight increase in IQ: 15 cases showed an increase in IQ of more than 5 points; in 12 cases IQ remained within 5 points of pre-test level; and in only 3 cases did IQ fall by more than 5 points.

Secondly, Broager and Olesen (1972) give an account of their experience with 63 cases of bilateral cingulectomy, on cases of intractable pain, depression and neuroses, claiming an 'excellent' or 'significant improvement' rate of 66 per cent. Thirdly, Mingrino and Schergna (1972) operated on 10 patients presenting violent and aggressive behaviour, all of whom were mentally retarded. Nine of these cases showed an immediate marked improvement in behaviour, but at followup (15 to 32 months) these good results had persisted in only 2 cases. They therefore conclude that so far as aggression is concerned, the cingulotomy has only a temporary therapeutic effect.

Before leaving the subject of cingulectomies, it is worth reiterating the fact that the 'frontal' syndrome is not often observed in cingulate cases, in spite of their close physical and anatomical connections, and in spite of a certain similarity in changes of mood, anxiety and aggression. This was pointed out as early as 1953, by Tow and Whitty in a very detailed (though not psychometric) analysis of 8 cingulectomy cases. They conclude that

> Our most important overall observation is that there has been little change in the total personality picture in these patients compared to the marked but transient behaviour changes seen in monkeys. In contrast also to what we can detect after a frontal leucotomy, although alterations occur in both instances in the sphere of social behaviour, the anterior cingulate subject shows nothing obviously unusual in his behaviour when one sees him, meets him or talks to him: to all intents and purposes he is normal'.

In sum, it seems that the cingulectomy reduces the personal experience of various negative and distressing mood states, as does the standard leucotomy, but without such pervasive adverse influences on personality. Unlike the amygdalectomy, the effect of cingulectomy on aggression is not pronounced, although in this respect the finding of Mingrino and Schergna (1972) needs replication.

Hypothalamic and thalamic lesions

Sano, Sekino and Mayanagi (1972) describe the effects of stimulating the hypothalamus by use of a needle electrode. In particular, there is an area in the posteromedial hypothalamus, described as the 'ergotropic triangle' which when stimulated led to a rise in blood pressure, tachycardia and pupillary dilation. It is this area that is excised during hypothalamotomy for violent and aggressive states. Sano et al. describe the outcome of the operation on a three-point rating scale — 'excellent', no need for observation, no violent or aggressive or restless episodes, calm and placid; 'good', calm and tractable but occasionally irritable; and 'unchanged'. The poverty of the assessment measures is, again, quite staggering, but for what they are worth the results are given in Table 6.5, which indicates a 95 per cent success rate. It can also be noted that of 22 cases who had uncontrollable seizures, 9 (41 per cent) showed a marked decrease in fit frequency.

The role of the hypothalamus in the maintenance of sexual performance has also received surgical attention from Roeder, Orthner and Muller (1972). They point out that after lesioning to the amygdaloid nucleus and pyriform cortex, cats and monkeys not only show calmness and fearlessness but also heightened sexual behaviour and responsiveness, that would cause males to mount both males and females and even other species. This behaviour they take to be a model of human sexual perversion, and since this hypersexuality can in animals

Table 6.5
Follow-up results of posteromedial hypothalamotomy (from Sano et al., 1972) at a follow up of from 2 to 8 years

	Over 15-years-old		Under 15-years-old	
	males	females	males	females
Excellent	8	5	3	4
Good	19	9	13	3
Unchanged	2	0	0	0

be reversed by supplemental destruction of the hypothalamic ventromedial nuclei, undertake the same operation in man: even though 'an attack on this region should . . . produce a general dampening effect on sexual function on a whole'.

Ten patients underwent the stereotaxic operation: 5 pedophiles; 4 homosexuals and 1 exhibitionist. Of these, 6 were claimed to have a complete cure, 1 a fair response, and 3 a poor response. A typical case history is given as follows

> *Case 2, male, 38 years*
> Educator with many years of pedophile tendencies. Dominant erotic objects, boys around 14 years of age. Compulsive homosexuality, uncontrollable, bordering on addiction.
> No pre-operative treatment.
> Hypothalamotomy on 7 May 1968. Followed up 3¼ years. Reduced sex drive. His former revulsion against women has completely disappeared. Enjoys company of young women (girl-friend). Meeting boys without experiencing any stimulation. Will take up his former profession. *Complete cure!*

The authors see the operation as a reasonable alternative to other possible treatments - prison, chemical and surgical castration - for the financial expense is low, libido gradually returns (presumably in a normally orientated direction) and the gonads continue to function. However, it is to be hoped that the operation will now be considered defunct in the light of improved sexual treatments, of the behaviour therapy variety.

In a second study concerning the effects on sex behaviour of stereotactic lesion to the hypothalamus, Dieckman and Hassler (1977) describe how they treated four violent sex offenders. Three were rapists and the fourth was an arsonist who was sexually motivated. All four voluntarily underwent lesioning to the sexual behaviour centres in the hypothalamus with the result that sex drive drastically diminished — so that both sex activity and sex problem reduced. The moral issues raised by the Roeder et al. (1972) and the Dieckman and Hassler (1977) studies are left to the reader to resolve. In my opinion, neither study has any scientific, experimental, clinical, neuropsychological, physiological, human or moral merit.

Turning from the hypothalamus to the thalamus, operations in this area have been aimed at a rather different set of behaviours subsumed under the name hyperresponsive syndrome (Andy and Jurko, 1972a), which is divided into three major groups: (a) hyperkinesia, (b) aggression, (c) patho-affect. The first two terms are self-explanatory, the last refers to neurotic mood disorders including depression, agitation, emotional lability and irritability.

Andy and Jurko (1972b) describe the use of the operation in 30 cases aged 6 to 49 years, and claim good results with 6 patients, fair results with 14 and poor results with 10 cases. The best clinical response was in cases of aggression, and the poorest in cases of patho-affect dysfunction.

As for the effects of thalamotomy on aspects of functioning not directly concerned with aggression, these have been assessed by Choppy, Zimbacca and Le Beau (1973). They compared left with right thalamotomy to find that the former has a more marked impact on a series of tests. After left thalamotomy, in 18 cases, verbal IQ fell ($p < .02$), self-criticism (related to neuroticism) reduced ($< .01$), verbal fluency fell ($p < 0.5$), score on a track tracing test fell ($p < .01$) and the depression and introversion scales on the MMPI fell ($p < .02$ and $p < .05$). After right thalamotomy (11 cases) there were only two significant changes in that writing speed increased and the MMPI Mf scale decreased ($p < .01$ and $p < .05$). There is an interesting suggestion, then, of a difference between thalamotomy to the dominant and non-dominant lobes, in a way that has not become apparent with cingulectomies, amygdalectomies or hypothalamotomies. This emphasises the need for multiple baseline research and a widening of measures to encompass characteristics above and beyond the target variable of aggression.

Overall, we see that the lack of consistent detailed psychological assessment of the effects of hypthalamotomies and thalamotomies does not allow us to differentiate these two operations from amygdalectomy. All three surgical interventions placate and calm behaviour, and in particular reduce aggression. There may be particular psychological sequelae to each of them, but until proper assessment measures are taken this fact will be obscured. For example, it cannot be claimed (as by Roeder et al.) that the hypothalamotomy has a special role regarding the reduction of libido, until it can be shown that the thalamotomy and amygdalectomy do not have such an effect.

The comment by Valenstein (1973) on the Roeder study seems very appropriate to repeat:

> clearly, this is an example of a group adopting a psychosurgical procedure based on an arbitrary selection from the total animal data available and then reporting their results in a completely inadequate form. No indication has been presented that these investigators have or intend to employ the type of behaviour testing necessary for an objective evaluation of post operative change.

Lesions to the temporal lobe

Many clinical observations have been made linking temporal lobe damage to depression, anxiety, withdrawal, aggression, disinhibition, personality change, irritability and so on, in addition to the vast experimental literature on cognitive processing abilities contained within the temporal lobes, including memory and language. It is the former type of function that will concern us here, and there are at least three reasons why these personality and emotional functions should be upset: (a) according to the damagedness hypothesis, any cortical lesioning is liable to have a detrimental influence on personality integrity, (b) the temporal lobes contain the amygdala and are an important link between the frontal cortex and the limbic system, with obvious implications for mood and emotional states, (c) the left temporal cortex has a special function regarding language, so that inasmuch as language is seen as an important controller of behaviour, its disturbance might lead to difficulties in behavioural and personality organisation and regulation (Blakemore, 1963).

The possibile regulatory and associative role of the temporal cortex has been outlined by Livingston and Escobar (1972).

> Thus, while the deep lying amygdala has received major emphasis as the dominant component of the basolateral limbic circuit in terms of aggressive behaviour, it seems likely that the anterior temporal cortex and its connections play a more sophisticated role — that of modulating emotional and behavioural activity related to sensory perception and its associated ideation and feeling. It seems reasonable to suggest that the anterior temporal cortex and its basolateral limbic connections may be involved in clinical disorders that can be visualised as malfunctions of perceptual and interpretive mechanisms.

There is some evidence that temporal lesions are more associated with personality dysfunctions than is any other cortical area. For example, Lishman (1968) in his investigation described earlier found that in 63 cases in which one or both of the temporal lobes were damaged, only 10 per cent had no psychiatric disability, 29 per cent had mild disability and no less than 61 per cent were severely disabled. This degree of association with disorder was higher than for frontal, parietal or occipital lesions. However, in Hécaen's (1964) series, also described earlier, temporal lesions seemed to have *less* disabling consequences for the individual than did frontal lesions. Here, 60 per cent of frontal cases suffered confusion and deterioration and 50 per cent suffered mood and character disturbances, whereas the respective figures for the temporally lesioned group were much less at 42.4 per cent and 22.2 per cent.

One thing is certain, though, that temporal lesions do severely affect the person, be this effect greater or less than with frontal lesions. The prevalence figures from Lishman and Hecaen have already been cited. To this we can add the extensive work of Falconer (1973) who reports the outcome of 100 temporal lobectomies administered for intractible temporal lobe epilepsy. Only 13 of his sample were psychiatically normal; 47 were diagnosed as psychopaths; 16 as psychotic; 27 showed extreme violence and aggression and 40 had received in-patient psychiatric clinic treatment. Even if we allow for the fact that the sample is highly selected (i.e. only includes those suitable for an operation), the figures are extremely high. Finally the work of Flor-Henry (1969), in outlining the relationship between left temporal lesions and psychosis, completes a fairly consistent picture.

Unfortunately, the amount of work directed towards refining our understanding (or even description) of these evident relationships has been minimal, especially in comparison with the memory and language literature.

McIntyre et al. (1976) try to define the personality effects of temporal lesions using various objective tests, including the Kagan matching familiar figures (MFF) test and the Davitz-Mattis metaphor (DMT) test. MFF is supposed to measure an individual's predisposition to respond quickly but erroneously thereby tapping an impulsivity-reflection trait that has some features in common with extraversion. The DMT test concerns the subject's ability to detect emotional meaning from verbal descriptions of common affective states, labelling 55 descriptions with either anger, anxiety, joy, love or sadness. The tests were given to three matched group of 11 left temporal cases, 11 right temporal cases and 12 controls (aged between 15 and 28 years, all right-handed).

The results for MFF and DMT are shown in Table 6.6. The finding on DMT, that left cases are worst of all at emotional labelling is understandable in the light of evidence of general emotional disturbances in left temporal cases. But the finding that left cases are more reflective on MFF is surprising in view of the supposed impulsivity and disinhibition that is clinically observed. Since the parameter of impulse control would seem an especially important one to assess given the supposed aggressiveness of left temporal cases, it is a pity that only one other study, by Dikman and Reitan (1974), utilises an acting-out or impulsivity index.

In this study, Dikman and Reitan match 15 aphasics to 15 brain injured controls, and administer the MMPI, which is scored in the ordinary way but with the addition of six composite indexes: (a) anxiety index (1.33 D + 1.00 Pt — .66 Hs — .66 Hy), (b) internalisation ratio (Hs + D + Pt/Hy + Pd + Ma), (c) expres-

Table 6.6
Comparison of left-lesioned, right-lesioned and controls on matching familar figures (MFF) and the metaphor test (DMT) (McIntyre et al., 1972)

	MFF			DMT
	Mean total time	Mean time to first response	Mean Errors	Mean non-consensual score
Left	118.58	88.27	10.36	17.73
Right	63.17	39.29	12.09	12.82
Controls	74.38	53.26	8.75	13.25
F	7.20	6.10		5.66
p	$<.01$	$<.01$	n.s.	$<.01$

sive-repressive index (L + K + Hy — Pd —Ma), (d) psychotic index (L + Pa + Sc — Hy — Pt), (e) cognitive slippage (Sc/Pt), (f) acting-out impulsivity index (Pd/Hy). The results are quite interesting in that by *t*-tests, the aphasic group comes out higher on Pd (psychopathic deviate) and Sc (schizophrenic) at the .005 level, very much in line with our expectations of the effects of temporal lesions.

There was also a trend for the aphasics to be higher on the neurotic triad (Hs + D + Hy) and on the psychotic triad (Pa + Pt + Sc), but these did not reach significance. Nor did any of the composite indexes reach significance, so, to the extent that the MMPI impulsivity index is tapping the same trait as MFF, the findings are contradictory. However, there is at least an indication that on two formal personality scores (Pd and Sc), left temporal lesions involving language are associated with deviant personality responses. There is, of course, one query about this study in that how did the language disturbed subjects cope with the language in the test itself? It is hoped that since the subjects were reportedly matched for IQ, this is not such a problem as it seems, especially if it were the case that verbal IQs were matched. However, it should be mentioned that in an earlier study by Reitan (Doehring and Reitan, 1960) in which 17 aphasics, 17 non-aphasic brain-damaged cases, and 17 normal controls were compared, differences on Pd and Sc were not found, but the groups were not so carefully matched as in the later study.

One final area to consider is the effect of the temporal lobectomy operation to reduce fitting. The nature of the original epileptogenic lesion is quite different to the nature of the surgical lesion; the former consisting, according to Falconer (1973), mainly of cortical lesions such as produced by medial temporal sclerosis (47 per cent of his cases) or cortical EEG foci relating to no specific observable lesion (25 per cent), whereas the surgical lesion encompasses more of the deep structure (see Fig. 6.10). Falconer (1973) when analysing his 100-case series, describes his standard resection as being performed *en bloc* including the hippocampus, the dorsolateral part of the amygdala, the parahippocamal gyrus and the uncus. In this case there is a more clear severing of the fronto-temporo-limbic circuit so that one would expect the effects on anxiety, depression, aggression and so forth, to be in line with cingulectomy results. There is only limited clinical data to support this as assessment procedures were designed only to measure changes in intellectual performance and fit frequency since it was not a 'psycho'-surgical operation. But Falconer does point out that of the 27 extremely aggressive cases he operated on, there was not only a very significant reduction in fit frequency in 22 (of at least 50 per cent) but also in 10 of them a very marked reduction in aggression.

A paper by Hill, Pond, Mitchell and Falconer (1957) gives a fairly detailed report of personality changes in a series of 31 temporal lobectomy cases reported earlier by Falconer et al. (1955). Four cases had dropped out by follow-up, and of the remaining 27, most had character disorders (e.g. psychopathic, schizoid,

Fig. 6.10 Temporal lobectomy operation (from Falconner et al., 1922). Stages of temporal lobectomy: *(a)* first stage, showing the line of incision in relation to sylvian vessels and Labbe's vein, *(b)* second stage, showing insula uncovered and temporal horn opened posteriorly, *(c)* third stage, showing temporal horn opened along its roof, exposing hippocampus in its floor with choroidal plexus lying above it, *(d)* representation of extent of removal of temporal lobe on completion of operation.

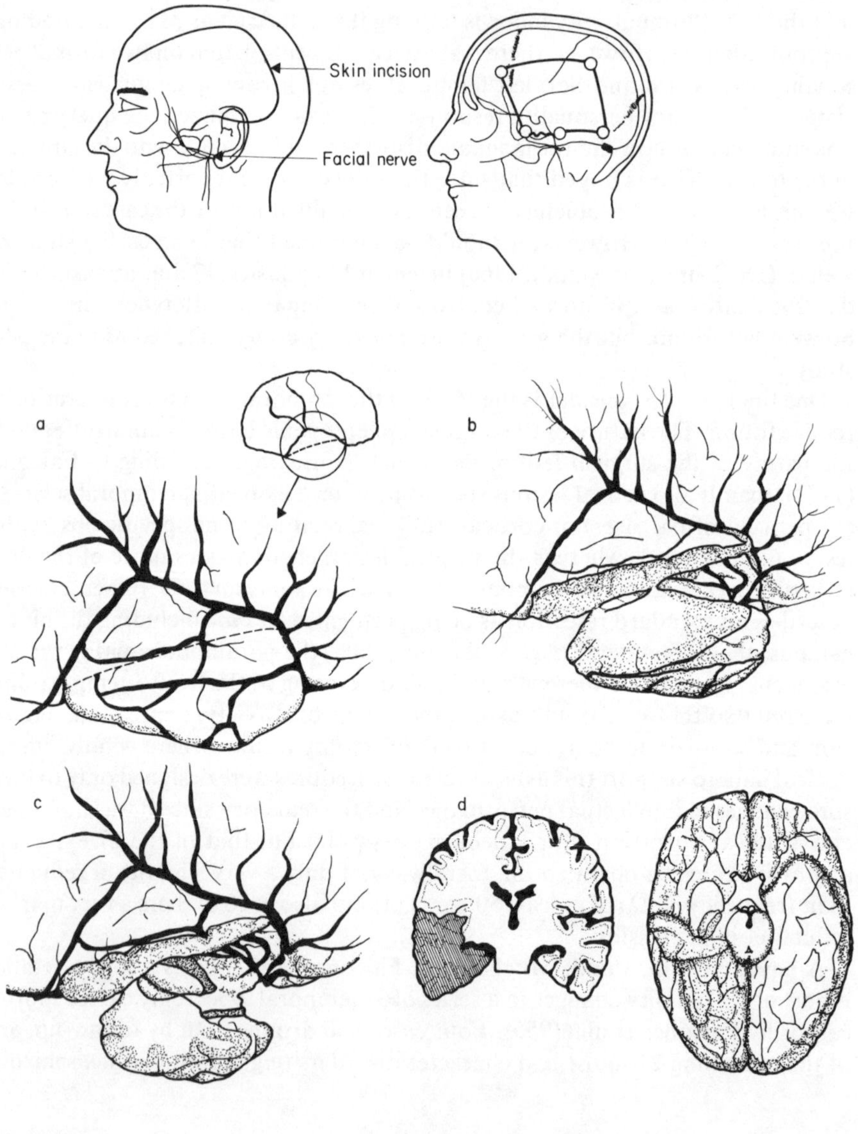

aggressive or sexually perverted). Of these, 10 suffered 'notoriously frequent outbursts' of aggression prior to the operation; afterwards 5 had 'no outbursts', 4 had 'occasional outbursts' and only 1 remained unchanged. The overall results for aggression are given in Table 6.7 where it is apparent that across all patients, 15 became less aggressive, 8 remained the same and 3 worsened.

In conclusion, it seems that we have surprisingly little evidence on which to base our understanding of the relationship that clearly exists between temporal damage and personality, affective and behavioural disturbances. This relationship cannot be modulated entirely by the amygdala since amygdalectomies do not either produce or relieve the psychiatric picture of temporal cases given by Lishman and Hécaen, although the amygdala may specifically regulate the aggressiveness noted in temporal cases. We are therefore left to suppose that damage to the cortex itself contributes to the clinical picture, but it is as yet impossible to delineate the relative contribution of cortical and amygdaloid damage.

Summary and synthesis

One way of conceptualising this rather difficult area of psychosurgery and the personality effects of accidental lesions, is to conceive of brain-personality relationships as being modulated by three related systems or tiers. System I concerns cortical processing and cortico-cortical fibres, and involves the perception and interpretation of events and situations, and the development of a strategy or plan of behavioural action: system II consists of the interchange of information between the cortex and limbic system, adding emotional colouring to perception and interpretation and influencing the emotive structure of behavioural plans and strategies; system III comprises the limbic circuits themselves which, on the basis of information from the cortex and from bodily, physical sensations and

Table 6.7
Changes in aggression (rated ++, + or 0) for 26 cases of temporal lobectomy (no. of *S*s in cells)

Pre-aggression rating	Post-aggression rate		
	++	+	0
++	1	4	5
+	3	5	6
0	0	0	2

states, determine an accurate picture of emotional status. The three systems are represented schematically in Fig. 6.11.

Lesions to any part of the three-tier system will therefore have an impact on personality along the following lines.

System I lesions

Such lesions will reduce the ability of the individual to perceive and interpret situational cues as to behaviour and inhibit his ability to formulate and choose between various plans of behaviour. This suggests he will lose an adaptive capacity such as might protect him from psychiatric illness in so far as he becomes less efficient at solving life problems and will exhibit a certain rigidity and/or inappropriateness of response. Further, the capacity of the cortex to control, inhibit, or override messages from the limbic system would be reduced, so that the individual is more likely to succumb to emotive stimuli and to respond impulsively to an emotive drive — another factor possibly detrimental to the psychiatric state of the person.

System II lesions

These will cause a disconnection syndrome (Geschwind, 1965) in that two systems that normally work in unison, the cortex and limbic systems, become divorced in their activity. If the two systems are not entirely disconnected, then, at the least, transmission between them will be unpredictable, distorted and misleading. Disruption for the individual will therefore be to the emotional sphere of behaviour and behaviour planning. Requests from the cortex for the limbic system to assist in the development of behavioural plans that have an emotional tone may remain unanswered; the cortex may make wrong assumptions about

Fig. 6.11 Three of the systems that regulate brain-personality relationships

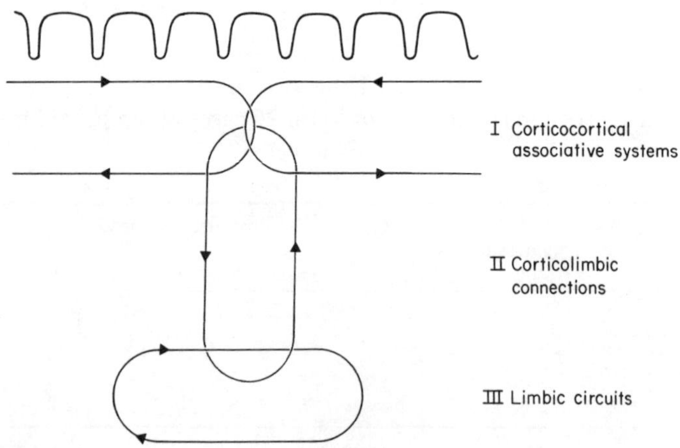

the affective state of the organism; and messages from the limbic system that would normally instigate appropriate associative processing and action do not arrive at the cortex. The state is one of desynchrony between perception, thought and action on the one hand, and psychophysiological emotion on the other.

System III lesions

These lesions will reduce the ability of the individual to synthesise emotional information from bodily states and sensations so that the individual will fail to appreciate affective states that actually exist, and may assume various states to exist that do not actually exist. Thus, whereas in the previous disconnection syndrome, the cortex may have to resolve actions in the absence of otherwise germane emotive information, in the present picture the cortex may do this and, in addition, act on falsely determined emotive states. In other words, the cortex not only has to deal with a *lack* of information but also the presence of *false* information. A further effect of limbic lesions will be to disturb the fine balance of activity between reciprocal and mutually exclusive 'centres', so that the activity in various circuits can become exaggerated, transmitting massive outbursts of activity to the cortex, which the cortex finds too strong to control or inhibit. This will cause the individual to suffer hyperresponsive, emotive behavioural outbursts.

We can now outline an explanation for the effects of psychosurgical and other lesions in the light of this model.

Standard leucotomy

This operation reduces the cortical processing capacity of the individual by a large amount thereby causing a decrement in intellectual and planning capacity, and a psychiatric picture as described by system I lesions above. In depriving the brain of its primary limbic projection area, the effect is that behaviour and experience tends to become affect-free. Since cortical control of limbic outpourings is obviously weakened, any affective behaviour that does occur is liable to be inappropriate or exaggerated.

Modified frontal operations

Here, surgery destroys much less brain tissue but still interrupt frontal-limbic connections. Because most of the cortex is preserved much less of a 'frontal' personality picture is obtained. The formation of behavioural strategies and their relative evaluation are performed adequately so that the individual can remain responsive to changes in circumstance, reasonably adaptable and flexible. The beneficial therapeutic effect of both these operations stems from the same fact of limbic messages failing to reach intact cortex. The apparent finding that behaviour is more emotion-free in the standard operation is probably not due to greater lesioning of frontal-limbic pathways, but due to the fact that there is more cortex available in the modified operation instance for the individual to use to infer appropriate emotion from external sources (i.e. situational cues). Similarly, because more of the cortex is preserved, any limbic messages that reach the cortex will be more appropriately interpreted and acted upon than is the case with the full lobotomy. One similarity between full and partial leucotomy is that they both alter general arousal by affecting the frontal-brain-stem loop, a factor that may account for the slight intellectual or performance losses noted in even the modified operation.

Cingulectomy

This comes close to being a disconnection syndrome. The cortex is left fully preserved and so there is no performance or intellectual deficit due to neuron loss or changes in the frontal-brain-stem arousal modulating system. The incongruities that should occur in behaviour, as discussed in relation to system II lesions above, are easily missed when we look at the abnormal cases who undergo the operation. For them, desynchrony is a desirable state of affairs; to be able to say that they should logically feel depressed or anxious or in pain, but that they actually have no such feeling, is therapeutically speaking a *beneficial* change, although it would be most unusual in an ordinary person.

Amygdalectomy

The effects here are a cross between the effects of lesions in both system II and system III, in that the amygdala is a part of the limbic system and also one of the major routes of access between the temporal cortex and the remainder of the limbic system. The amygdaloid nucleus has some special link with aggressiveness, and in many violent cases abnormal EEG spiking is to be observed here. Therefore its destruction relieves the temporal cortex of the task of trying to control or inhibit unusually exaggerated messages from the amygdala. Whether there are any other emotional sequelae to the operation, particularly of the disconnection variety that we would predict, is unknown because of the poor assessment techniques used in studies.

Hypothalamotomy and thalamotomy

Both these operations seem to be direct attempts to modify the activity in various limbic circuits that appear to have gone out of control. This type of operation, i.e. one that attempts to deal with a specific, identifiable circuit contributing to the organisation of just one type of behaviour (it could be eating, drinking, sexual behaviour and so on) may well have the most circumscribed impact of all on personality, since the other surgical procedures sever pathways that may subserve a whole variety of functions. Future psychosurgery methods will probably be concerned more and more with the destruction of highly specialised areas, rather than with the destruction of highly non-specialised areas such as the frontal lobes.

Before leaving the topic of brain lesions there is one loose end to tie up: how these results relate to formal organic theories of personality, i.e. Eysenck's and Gray's modification to it. There are three aspects to consider.

The corticoreticular model of extraversion (Eysenck)

The studies reported here do not bear directly on this general model which concerns the state of the cortex as a whole, for we have only considered particular lesions. However, it must be pointed out that changing arousal by frontal lesions does not seem to cause an increase in extraversion. The immediate question now must be why depressant drugs such as alcohol cause extravert behaviours by modifying arousal, whereas frontal lesions do not, even though they too modify arousal. The most immediate answer must be that in the frontal case, cortical tissue — often a very considerable amount — has been destroyed. The comparison, therefore, between drug effects and frontal effects is an unfair one. As we saw in chapter 5, cortical damage leads to a considerable disorganisation in personal and interpersonal functioning that can swamp any 'delicate' effects of slight changes in arousal. The notion of generalised cortical tone being at the heart of extraversion, is not, therefore; weakened by the frontal leucotomy findings.

The orbital cortex-limbic system-reticular model of extraversion (Gray)

The orbital cortex part of this model must now be firmly rejected since lesions to the cingulate gyrus that divorce the orbital cortex from the limbic system do not increase extraversion but decrease neuroticism (although there is some conflicting evidence, see Walsh, 1977, and Bailey et al. 1977). If Gray is correct in claiming that extraverts are less susceptible to punishment, then the sensitivity to punishment system he describes must be able to operate adequately without the superordinate control of the orbital frontal cortex. The onus is upon Gray to rework his model accordingly.

The limbic-ARAS model of neuroticism (Eysenck)

It is clear from the papers reviewed here that activity within the limbic system is important to many aspects of neurotic behaviour. Since the limbic system can be activated by the ARAS, then the limbic-ARAS loop that Eysenck describes is self-evidently important. However, it is only part of the story. Severing cortical-limbic connections has been shown to reduce neurotic anxiety, depression and so forth (and, indeed, actual questionnaire measures of N), and so this facet of connectivity between limbic circuits and cortical circuits needs encompassing as has been achieved in Gray's model. If we view these disconnection operations as relieving the cortex of the task of controlling emotional limbic outpourings, and view low N as the ability to cognitively override, control or modify emotional impulses from the limbic system, then it would seem that low N is just as much a 'processing' capacity as some measurable state of the hardware. Of course the two will be related since greater activity in the limbic system would presumably make such 'processing' more difficult.

7 Individual differences in the organisation of cortical processing

So far, emphasis has been placed on actual or hypothetical properties of the nervous system, and on certain fixed physical neural connections. If we consider this to be the 'hardware' side of processing — the equipment at our disposal to complete tasks imposed on us by the environment — then we have not yet considered 'software' aspects, i.e. the programming, or how information is shuttled about the system, how information is collected, sampled, or combined, and so on. Most of these latter processing aspects are out of the scope of this chapter, since they really lie within the realm of pure experimental psychology, rather than neuropsychology. But there is almost bound to be an interplay between the strategy of task solution and the nature of the available equipment. The following three topics touch on this relationship between structure and function.

Redundancy in neural processing

The concept of redundancy is central to the areas of visual, auditory and semantic perception, for to a great extent it governs the intelligibility of the stimulus or message — a specific stimulus when embedded within an associated (i.e. redundant) context, such as a particular word when placed in a sentence, is more readily perceived and understood. There is a trade-off against total information content in that a high-redundant message cannot carry as much information as a low-redundant message. The latter is more 'risky' since there are fewer internal cues to meaning and hence a greater probability of misapprehension (see Garner, 1962 and Fig. 7.1).

The degree of redundancy in brain processing is not a fixed quantity, as Pribram (1968) points out. When the brain carries a signal, it is not normally along just a single neuron route, but across many, so that if one neuronal route fails through physical interruption or excessive channel noise, the signal may still reach its destination via the remaining fibres. But the point Pribram makes is that the number of fibres that carry a message is variable, not just by chance, but by deliberate design at the order of the associative cortex. Hence a degree of control over input can be achieved by the cortex (Spinelli and Pribram, 1966), and changes in the state of the cortex will affect channel redundancy (Dewson et al., 1966; Spinelli and Pribram, 1966).

Pribram postulates that this dimension of redundancy is one along which people vary.

On the input side, redundancy *reduction* is involved when interest and sen-

Fig. 7.1 Schematic representation of high and low redundancy in processing

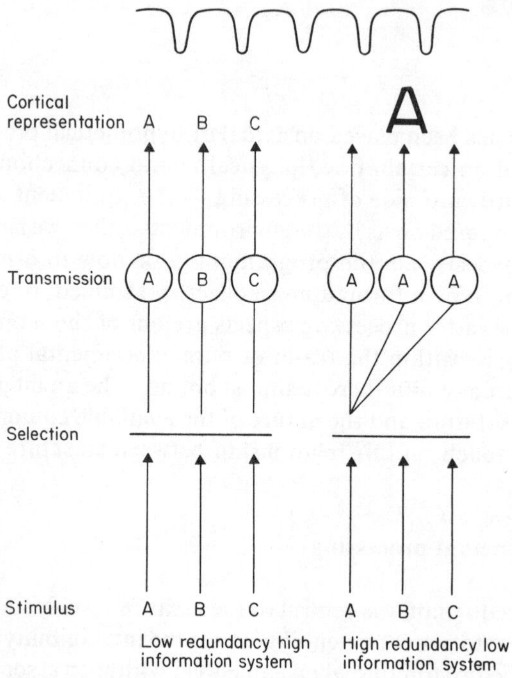

> sory *participation* are called forth: redundancy *enhancement* helps *focus and restrict* the organism's sensory interaction with the situation. The two processes are ordinarily balanced, for they converge on the same input mechanism, even on some of the same cells in the mechanism. (Spinelli and Pribram 1967, pp. 143-9, his italics).
>
> It is likely that the adjustment of this balance differs in different individuals in different situations. (Pribram, 1968)

Although there is no direct study relating changes or differences in this redundancy balance to human behaviour or personality, Pribram is able to patch up an argument as follows: (a) frontal leucotomy changes individuals towards the extravert end of an introversion-extraversion dimension, (b) removal of frontal lobe tissue leads to a reduction of redundancy in input channels, and therefore (c) differences in redundancy can explain differences in performance between introverts and extraverts.

The evidence may not be appealing, especially after the earlier analysis of frontal lesions, but the resultant conclusion is intriguing. Is the introvert's desire for caution, sameness and preference for predictability paralleled by a highly redundant processing system that is equally as safety conscious and restrictive? Is the extravert's quest for novelty, change and desire for wide sensory involvement paralleled by low-redundancy processing that admits all kinds of extra sensory stimulation?

To see compatibility or congruence between measures at such disparate levels of analysis may be too optimistic, yet there are other ways that the notion of redundancy may be important, particularly in predicting the effects of brain damage. If an individual typically carries *x* amount of information on a total of *y* fibres, it is clear that if some fibres are lost through damage (and there are no others available to replace them), then the ratio *x*:*y* can only be maintained by reducing the amount of information carried in proportion to the percentage of fibres lost. This will maintain the habitual redundancy level but cause information to be lost at some earlier selection stage. The alternative is to assign fewer fibres per bit of information, a strategy that will attempt to carry the same load by decreasing redundancy but risk losing information by channel or transmission noise. After brain damage, then, both strategies will lead to information loss either through intentional filtering or by transmission distortion. But the types of loss in the two cases would be quite different. Information loss in the former instance would be predictable — assuming that the individual would filter out non-pertinent, less relevant information as being less important to carry. In the second case, information loss would be across all types of information and less predictable, assuming a random distribution of noise of equal mean for all fibres.

If we argue along these lines, we can develop the prediction that a given lesion will affect introverts and extraverts in different ways, in the same way, for example, that response to brain damage is influenced by the 'goodness' or 'poorness' of pre-morbid personality (Lishman, 1968).

Brainedness

Another area of research which suggests that a particular lesion will have differential effects governed by the individual's current mode of processing information comes from the work of Buffery (1975; Buffery and Gray, 1972). Buffery's concept of brainedness refers to the extent that neural processes are lateralised into one or other of the cerebral hemispheres, e.g. the degree of left hemisphere dominance for verbal information (verbal brainedness) or the degree of right dominance for visual-spatial tasks (spatial brainedness).

Buffery (1975) reports an experiment in which 200 normal *S*s (100 male, aged 18 to 25) had to say whether a pair of stimuli projected via a tachistoscope, to either the left or right hemisphere, were 'same' or 'different'. One-half of the stimuli were to be matched on a semantic basis (two monosyllabic nouns having the same or different meaning) and the other half were to be matched visually (two non-verbalisable spatial stimuli that were or were not identical). According to their performance on each of these tasks, *S*s were categorised as 'strongly left-brained', 'left-brained', 'mixed-brained', 'right-brained' or 'strongly right-brained'. Hence each *S* obtained a score on both verbal brainedness and on spatial brainedness, as displayed in Table 7.1.

Several points are readily apparent: (a) the rule of thumb stating that verbal processing is carried out by the left brain, and spatial processing by the right brain is *only* a rule of thumb, because 40.5 per cent of *S*s do not have the pattern of (+L, +R), a finding not accounted for by the sample having a high percentage of left-handers (only 8 per cent were left-handed), (b) in normal *S*s one hemisphere can predominate for both kinds of task, found in 11 cases, or 5.5 per cent, (c) the relationship between degree of verbal and degree of spatial brainedness is not that of a perfect correlation, since 23.5 per cent of *S*s did not fall along the left to right diagonal of table, (d) women are more strongly lateralised than men since 71 per cent of females shown the +L, +R pattern in comparison with 48 per cent of men.

It is this last finding of all, the finding of a sex difference in lateralisation, that is most relevant here for it can go some way to explaining why women are better than men at language tasks, and vice versa for spatial skills (Buffery and Gray 1972). The assumption is that verbal tasks are better undertaken by a brain that is more tightly organised into specialised centres, whereas spatial skills require a more diffuse brain organisation. Buffery and Gray suggest that the sex difference is evident right from birth and may have a genetically determined structural basis; in this respect Witelson and Pallic (1973) found the temporal planum (approximately Wernicke's area) to be larger in female than male neonates, indicating the former to be more 'prepared' for left dominance in language.

If there is this important gender difference in brain processing whereby men are more likely to utilise both hemispheres when analysing information, can it

Table 7.1

Distribution of 100 men and 100 women on scores of verbal and spatial brainedness (VB and SB)

	Women, VB					Men, VB				
SB	+L	L	M	R	+R	+L	L	M	R	+R
+R	71	1	1	1	0	48	3	2	3	1
R	4	7	0	0	1	6	11	1	0	0
M	4	1	1	0	0	8	3	7	0	0
L	2	1	0	3	0	2	0	2	3	0
+L	0	0	0	0	2	0	0	0	0	0

predict or account for any of the personality differences apparent between males and females?

The most promising place to start would be to try and draw a parallel between the articulated (female) v. global (male) mode of neural processing as outlined above and Witkin's (1965) concept of an articulated v. global dimension of personality and cognitive functioning. This dimension is assessed by various measures such as the body adjustment test in which the *S* sits in a chair that can be tilted within a room that can also be tilted, the task being for the *S* to estimate his angle of lean as accurately as possible. The field-independent person, who articulates internal from external cues, will perform better than the field-dependent person who relies on visual cues from the surrounding room, i.e. who processes in a more global fashion. Another test is the embedded figure test where *S*s have to detect a simpel figure hidden within a complex design. The field-dependent, global thinker will perform the worse.

It would now be conveniently neat if women were (a) articulated in neural organisation and (b) articulated, or field independent, on Witkin's personality dimension — and men were the converse in both respects. Such congruence does not, however, seem to exist, because a small but consistent sex difference in favour of higher field independence for men has been found by several authors (Andrieux, 1955; Bennett, 1956). But there is some confusion here in that field dependence is associated with high spatial IQ scores on block design, picture completion and object assembly (Karp, 1963). This suggests that men, who score higher on these tests (see Buffery and Gray, 1972), are field dependent or global processors.

Therefore, although the evidence is mixed it would probably be premature to reject the notion of a correlation between Witkin's psychological differentiation and Buffery's brainedness, especially since such a relationship might tie in with Eysenck's dimension of extraversion. Eysenck (1968), p. 117) sees field dependence and independence as 'closely' pertaining to extraversion and introversion respectively - dependence being viewed as a measure of the degree of perceptual determination by external percepts, a feature of extravert processing. As far as the previously noted sex difference is concerned, a finding of males being higher on field dependence would then be congruent with the male's higher scores on extraversion.

Extraversion has now been mentioned in relation to both redundancy and brainedness. It can be seen, in fact, that these two concepts are not wholly unrelated. If we consider a hemisphere in a low-lateralised subject, it will be attempting to process both verbal and spatial information, which is equivalent to saying that it is a low-redundant system which processes a greater amount or diversity of information.

There is now a cluster of dimensions — maleness, extraversion, field dependence, low brainedness and low redundancy — that seem to be conceptually related, and which await further detailed empirical investigation.

Perceptual moment hypothesis

A further example of the possible interplay between structure and function, or psychological and neural processing, concerns the perceptual moment. Although there are many variants of the perceptual moment theory, they all centre around the idea that processing at the cortical level is discontinuous; that the brain does not attempt to make sense of each of the billions of impulses that reach the cortex each second but instead takes an average of all events within a previous interval. The interval across which neural messages are averaged is referred to as the 'moment'. Neural events that occur within the same moment are not discriminated but pooled together. Only impulses that arrive in separate moments can be distinguished as separate.

There were several early pointers to such quantification or discontinuity, as outlined by Harter (1967) and Shallice (1964): (a) if two stimuli occur at less than a critical time they are perceived as simultaneous, (b) subjective estimates of the frequency of rapidly occurring stimuli do not bear a simple relationship to objective frequency, (c) corrective movements in motor control tasks are not smoothly continuous but consist of rapid small jerks in a manner that cannot be entirely accounted for by muscular limitations, (d) if two stimuli are presented in rapid succession the latter can mask the former, (e) a stimulus can appear to move fluidly through space if presented successively in different spatial locations (i.e. apparent movement), (f) a rapidly discontinuous (flickering) signal is perceived as constant in a way that is not wholly consistent with any peripheral processing limitations, (g) a bright visual signal presented for a short time has the same subjective brightness as a duller signal presented for longer ($I \times t = k$) in a manner not accounted for entirely by retinal phenomena, (h) when subjects are asked to tap as rapidly as possible, tapping rate is not constant but taps are clustered together in bursts, (i) if speech is rapidly switched from ear to ear then eventually language perception breaks down.

All of these observations gave a time for the perceptual moment of about 100 ms, or at least somewhere between 50 and 200 ms, dependent on the individual and the task. The basic phenomenon of the perceptual moment has stood up to fairly rigorous laboratory definition. For example, Kristofferson (1967) developed the paradigm in which (a) a light and tone would start simultaneously but the light would be switched off t seconds before the tone, and (b) the light and tone would both start and finish simultaneously. The *S* would be presented with A and then B (or vice versa) and be required to say in which instance the stimuli stopped at different times. Kristofferson showed that the probability of being correct stayed at zero for very low values of t before rapidly rising to one. He explained his results by saying that attention can only switch from one channel to another at the end of a quantum period (i.e. moment), so that if signals in the auditory and visual channels cease within one quantum or moment, they will be seen as ending simultaneously, since attention cannot switch in time to make the proper channel comparison. Allport (1968) further shows that fairly sophisticated predictions can be made using the quantum idea, as he examines an apparent movement phenomenon.

As for an explanation of why the brain needs to operate on a discontinuous time basis, there seems to be at least two good reasons. First, to reduce the information load on brain processing, as mentioned earlier. Secondly, as a means of coding or labelling information in terms of time of occurrence, assuming that information can be temporally tagged in this way. This would mean that different brain areas would be able to operate on the same time base.

Explanations of the physical basis of the quantum initially centred upon the α rhythm — that this rhythm corresponded to a scanning and averaging of cortical potentials (see Mackay, 1953; Surwillow, 1964; Harter, 1967). For example, Harter develops the idea of an excitability cycle of the cortex in which cortical thresholds vary rhythmically, in step with the α rhythm which is seen as the result of a large number of neurons having synchronous membrane potentials. Such a simple view can be well discredited for it is apparent that the moment is not as straightforward as at first sight. For example, Oatley (1969) indicates that the moment is not a static quantity, ticking away like an internal clock, but can be modified by the nature of the events themselves. In particular, he describes how moments can be triggered by a stimulus.

Many of the complexities of cortical discontinuity theory are taken up by Shallice (1964) who concludes that we need to envisage at least two types of moment or, as he describes them, accumulators. These are firstly specific accumulators attached to neural systems, channels or modalities that can function independently of each other if necessary, and can have properties adapted to particular

Fig. 7.2 A model of the perceptual moment system (from Shallice, 1962)

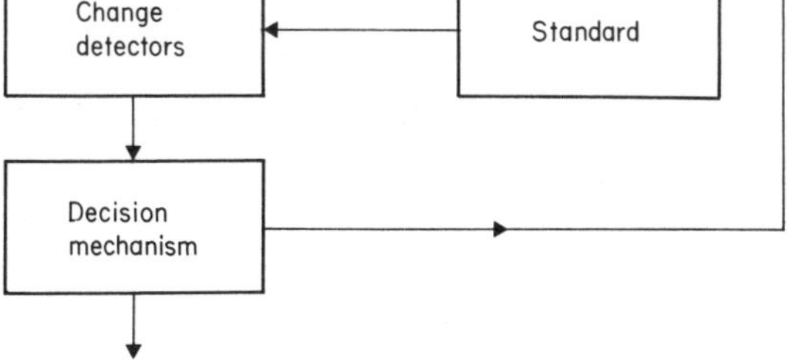

task demands, and secondly, an overall, co-ordinating accumulator. This general accumulator would receive input from all receptors. When input accumulates to a certain fixed level, its discharge is triggered which in turn triggers the discharging of all the specific accumulators, at which point, with every accumulator empty, the cycle starts afresh (Fig. 7.2).

A relationship is now apparent between the purely psychological theory of discontinuity, and an organic substrate centring upon the reticular activating system. When an individual is alert or aroused, the RAS is in a greater state of activity so that the reticular accumulator reaches its fixed discharge point sooner. Hence the perceptual moment becomes shorter and brain processing more exact or efficient, until a point of reticular activation is reached at which the moment is so short that the brain is overloaded with information (i.e. output from accumulators), causing performance to drop. This seems to be quite an accurate statement of the Yerkes-Dodson law, and of the performance difference between extraverts and introverts. The conceptualisation of extraverts as having slowly filling accumulators (at the risk of making them sound like second-hand car batteries) may link with findings such as higher sensory and pain thresholds of the extravert, the errors of inertia (i.e. lack of rapid change detection) in flying, the preference or search for additional stimulation, and so on. Although some results — such as CFF — may be difficult to square with the hypothesis of differences in perceptual moment size, it would seem worth while to test it specifically, perhaps by comparing extraverts and introverts on the task described by Kristofferson (1967), from which the size of the moment can be estimated.

8 Towards a neuropsychology of personality

The first issue to be taken up here will be that of measurement, for models and measurement must of necessity travel hand in hand. The measurements and the observations that are made are the building blocks of any model, so that however potentially important or crucial a certain element might be for a model, it can have no existence unless noted or assessed in some way. Ideally the model once constructed will cause a development of measurement technique and an increase of breadth, so as to eventually encompass any important but previously missed elements. In short, what we look for determines the model, and the model determines what we look for. In another area of neuropsychology, for example, psycholinguistic models have caused new observations to be made in aphasic patients, and extensive evaluation of aphasics has led to considerable modification in performance orientated linguistic models (see Goodglass and Blumstein, 1973).

Currently used measures of personality and their limitations

The ways in which behaviour has been measured in the studies reviewed collapse into various categories each with their own advantages and limitations

Personality dimensions

As assessed by properly standardised questionnaires (Leyton, HDQ, MPI, EPI and MMPI), such dimensions have been rarely used in studies of brain and behaviour or the effects of brain damage. When they have been used the results have often been highly informative, such as when Levinson and Meyer (1965) found that frontal cases did not have elevated E scores or when Kelly (1973) found a decrease in N after cingulate lesioning. The main advantages of standardised questionnaires are that they normally come with a surrounding body of theoretical and empirical knowledge that greatly facilitates the interpretation of results, and that they provide a shorthand description of the subject's behaviour. In practice there seem to be two main limitations. The first is that many subjects cannot complete questionnaires properly, such as the subnormal patients operated on by Narabayashi et al. (1963) or various aphasic groups. The second is that behavioural description from questionnaires is highly generalised and cannot be tailored towards specified features of behaviour change. In the MPI or EPI for example, only one or two items pertain to aggression and impulse control that are the most frequent target behaviours of psychosurgical operations.

Pseudo-dimensions

These seem to abound in the area of brain and personality. The most obvious is the rating of 'improvement' along some kind of 3-, 5- or whatever-point scale (e.g. Ballantine et al., 1967; Laitinen and Vilki, 1972; Kelly et al., 1973). There is no evidence ever presented that the concepts underlying 'improvement' are scalable or that the resultant scale is unifactorial. So many features go towards defining 'improvement' that the scales often completely fail to describe any particular subject (e.g. Narabayaski et al., 1963), a problem that is not resolved simply by the presentation of a few 'typical' case histories. Another clear example of a pseudo-dimension is the psychiatric rating scale, such as the 'mild' and 'severe' psychiatric disability scale used by Lishman (1968).

That this type of rating can never be a true scale is apparent from the fact that a psychotic illness would be seen as severe, and most neurotic ones are mild, whereas all the evidence suggests that psychotic illness and neurosis are *separate* entities and cannot be aligned in this manner (Eysenck and Eysenck, 1976). Such psychiatric ratings may be useful to give a rough glimpse of the individual's ability to cope with living, but it would be more useful to give such a description in a more articulated manner; ability to make friends, ability to handle close personal relationships, ability to manage emotions, ability to function during stressful crises, and so on. A start in this direction has been made by Post et al. (1968), even though their data base was very poor, as discussed previously.

Reports of specific behaviours and case histories

The use of case history descriptions has been a powerful tool in physical medicine, in which the medical model of illness (aetiology-symptoms-prognosis) applies. It is not, therefore, surprising that the case history has been used as an assessment tool in the field of psychosurgery, which is essentially a physical procedure. But inasmuch as the physical treatment has a psychological target, we must move from the 'case history method' to the 'single case study method' with all its scientific implications (Yule and Hemsley, 1977). At the very least this implies that the recording of data should be systematic; most surgical wards would use a fit chart or complete a blood pressure chart, for example, but very few have ever kept aggression charts or nature of activity charts or mood charts in the same way. It is not enough to rely on nurses' notes that may be jotted down hurriedly at the daily handover period. This haphazard reporting of specific behaviours relies too much on what a particular nurse, or doctor, or relative happens to think is important or happens to notice or, happens to define as aggression, or anxiety or depression.

Laboratory task performance

It goes almost without saying that the performance of subjects under laboratory conditions on standard tasks is essential to the furtherance of knowledge regarding brain and personality relationships, and the work of Petrie (1952; Petrie and Le Beau, 1956) and Tow (1955) is to be applauded. However, one should not rely too much on laboratory task performance as an adequate predictor of subjects' real life, overt performance. In another area of neuropsychology, memory, Bennett-Levy (1978) has shown enormous discrepancies in functioning between laboratory and real-life settings. In addition, such tasks should not be solely relied on to describe overt behaviour in the molar sense. Tow, for example, did not use a single questionnaire measure of personality to back up his laboratory findings; there is much more to extraversion than doing Porteus mazes.

Currently used measures of brain

With regard to measures of personality, the problem is not so much a lack of sophistication of assessment techniques — many excellent and extensive books have been written on the theory and method of assessment (e.g. Wiggins, 1973) — but more a lack of its application. With the brain, however, our main limitation is upon what we are *able* to measure. At present, our measures centre on the establishment of various dimensions and on the examination of specific lesions.

The measurement of brain according to dimensions is seen in a variety of ways:

balance of excitation-inhibition
amount of 'excitability substance'
degree of activity in corticoreticular loop
degree of activity in limbic-reticular loop
reactivity of neurons
redundancy in processing
size of perceptual moment
amount of tissue destroyed
degree of lateralisation

Of these, and others, many present enormous measurement problems. For example, degree of activity in a corticoreticular loop can only be measured by continuous monitoring via implanted electrodes, techniques we are only just beginning to work towards in animals; redundancy in processing, if it is to be measured at the organic level, would involve single cell recording, an even more difficult feat; and 'amount of excitability substance' involves its biochemical identification and measurement *in situ*. We are forced to continue, then, analysing brain according to an individual's performance on tasks whose underlying mechanisms we claim to understand, and to continue with the use of hypothetical constructs that we consider reasonable so far as prevailing evidence admits.

The measurement of brain by the presence of a lesion is obviously far closer to organic matters, but none the less without problems. Naturally or accidentally occurring lesions are difficult to define in extent and location (although the EMI scanner is helping out in this respect). Even stereotaxic surgical lesions are very large in comparison to the minute complexity of the brain. There are around 22 different nuclear groups within the amygdala (Isaacson, 1975) for example, all of which are wiped out by amygdalectomy. Therefore we have no clues as to the contribution of each of these groups to human behaviour and personality. Once again, improvement in the measurement of lesioning must attend technical advance particularly in the direction of smaller and more precisely aimed stereotaxic lesions.

New approaches to the measurement of emotion

The model presented in chapter 7 conceptualised changes in affective behaviour after brain lesions as related to the damage of one of three systems: corticocortico associative fibres that place emotive information within a total behavioural context; corticolimbic fibres that form the liaison network between cortex and limbic system; and limbic circuits in which affective information is generated. It was suggested that the clinical benefit derived from surgical procedures aimed at reducing the experience of negative affect (anxiety, pain, aggression, depression, etc.) should be seen as just one aspect of an overall change in the affect system. This suggests that future trends in the measurement of psychosurgical effects in this area should centre upon describing changes in the affect system as a whole — not just the primary unwanted target behaviours. Three types of measurement should be used.

Scale measures

These should of course continue in usage, to include standard personality questionnaires like the direction of hostility questionnaire (Caine et al., 1967), the manifest anxiety scale, and the neuroticism scale; also to include various other rating scales such as daily mood-adjective checklists and ratings; and finally to encompass direct observation schedules to be completed by others close to the patient.

Direct observation in standard situations under laboratory conditions

One of the problems of assessing the effects and side effects of brain lesions is that the behaviour is evaluated in a second-hand manner using information provided by others who have seen the patient behaving. Not only is this a gross measure, not refined enough to comment on the affect system as a whole, but it is open to all kinds of observer biases too numerous to mention. One alternative is to employ the same strategy as used in social skills studies (Argyle, 1969), which is to observe directly the individual under laboratory conditions during standard situations, recording the results on videotape for later scoring and blind rating. We now have a sample of behaviour permanently recorded which we can examine at leisure for changes or disturbance in the minutiae of affective detail. In cases where the cortical-limbic fibres have been severed for example, we would be particularly interested in the extent to which normal affect appears in the individual's behaviour. Has the range of expression in the voice been altered? What is the range of facial expression? Do facial and vocal emotive expressions match? Does the individual show warmth and empathy and consideration in conversation? Are there incongruencies between what the subject says or does and the facial, vocal or postural emotion displayed? Further, the laboratory situation can be altered to assess the patient's response to being rebuked, or to having self-esteem attacked, or to assess the response to frustration in a task.

Laboratory tasks

There are various laboratory tasks or phenomena that depend on affective processing. In cases where the affective system is expected to be changed, these tasks should be included in the test battery as surely as the WAIS or memory tests. These tasks may include: (a) perceptual defence (Dixon, 1971) or delayed reaction time to high-affectively toned stimuli such as taboo words — are these phenomena still apparent in subjects if the cortex is denied access to the limbic system? (b) labelling of emotions — here McIntyre et al. (1976) asked subject to label the emotional content of written passages, but one could add to this the interpretation of facial expression or vocal expression, (c) semantic differential — if the individual becomes more affect-free it could change their whole evaluation of affectively toned words such as 'kill', 'rape' or 'smash', suggesting that the rating of such words on a semantic differential type task would be a useful way of detecting change or abnormality, (d) humour — appreciation of jokes and so on has already been included in some batteries (e.g. Tow, 1958) and should stay, with the possible addition of the appreciation of different types of humour, (e) *in vivo* phobic tasks — there are two points here. Firstly a lesion that, say, reduces the appreciation of pain or anxiety may facilitate a more widely spread increase in approach behaviour towards previously declared phobic stimuli. Secondly, such a change in phobic behaviour may appear as desynchrony, i.e. dissociation between the elements of cognition, behaviour and physiological responsiveness in fear behaviour (Rachman and Hodgson, 1974).

New approaches to the meaning of personality

Throughout this book it has been the implicit assumption that personality is organised into traits: an individual's position on some behavioural dimension will predict his performance in many different settings. This dimensional or trait approach towards personality theory and personality assessment has been severely criticised over the last 10 years or so by the 'situationalism' school, or 'antitrait' theorists, largely led by Mischel (1968, 1969, 1973, 1977). The basic thesis of the antitrait theorists is that people are simply not as consistent as they, or we, appear to be; that we show much more flexibility of behaviour from situation to situation than we give ourselves credit for; or, as Hogan, De Soto and Solano (1977) state, in its extreme form 'personality traits are best viewed not as properties of individuals but as value judgements placed on actors by observers'. Because of the actual lack of consistencies in individuals, the validity coefficients of standard personality tests rarely reach even .30, so that behaviour must be considered as largely a function of situational parameters including various constraints, reinforcement contingencies, and expectations established during prior experience of the same situation (Mischel, 1968). The extreme position, i.e. complete situationalism denying all person variables, is in fact indefensible given that *some* consistency *does* exist. Therefore most personality theorists now walk some kind of middle path, that of interactionalism, which is a personality x situation model (Endler and Magnusson, 1976; Hogal et al., 1977; Mischel, 1977).

The relevance of this newer approach is that it encourages the view that personality consists of *cognitive processes*, and therefore makes the area more compatible with other neuropsychological topics such as language and memory that also involve cognitive processing. This is made clear if we consider the definition of personality offered by Mischel (1977):

> The image is one of the human being as an active, aware problem solver, capable of profiting from an enormous range of experiences and cognitive capacities, possessing great potential for good or ill, actively constructing his or her psychological world, and influencing the environment but also being influenced by it in lawful ways — even if the laws are difficult to discover and hard to generalise. It views the person as so complex and multifaceted as to defy easy classification and comparisons on any single or simple common dimension, as multiply influenced by a host of interacting determinants, as uniquely organised on the basis of prior experiences and future expectations, and yet as rule-guided in systematic, potentially comprehensible ways that are open to study by the methods of science. It is an image that has moved a long way from the instinctual drive-reduction models, the static global traits, and the automatic stimulus-response bonds of traditional personality theories.

The active, evaluative, predictive and planning capacities alluded to obviously have much in common with the view of personality offered by Miller, Gallanter and Pribram (1960) as they discuss the structure of behaviour, or with Luria's (1966) notions concerning the regulatory function of the human frontal lobes. Some of the most important points concerning the cognitive-situation control of behaviour are expressed in Fig. 8.1. We can now consider in more detail some of the ramifications of this model for a neuropsychological theory of personality and for the types of measures that should be employed for the elaboration of brain-personality relationships. There seem to be three main processes to consider: the evaluation of the elements that go towards defining the situation, the formulation of alternative plans, and the relative evaluation of plans.

Subjective evaluation/interpretation of situational elements

Constructing a subjective impression of the situation, attaching personal meaning to the 'objective' definition, is the primary stage in the situational determina-

Fig. 8.1 Representation of the situation's impact on behaviour according to cognitive personality models

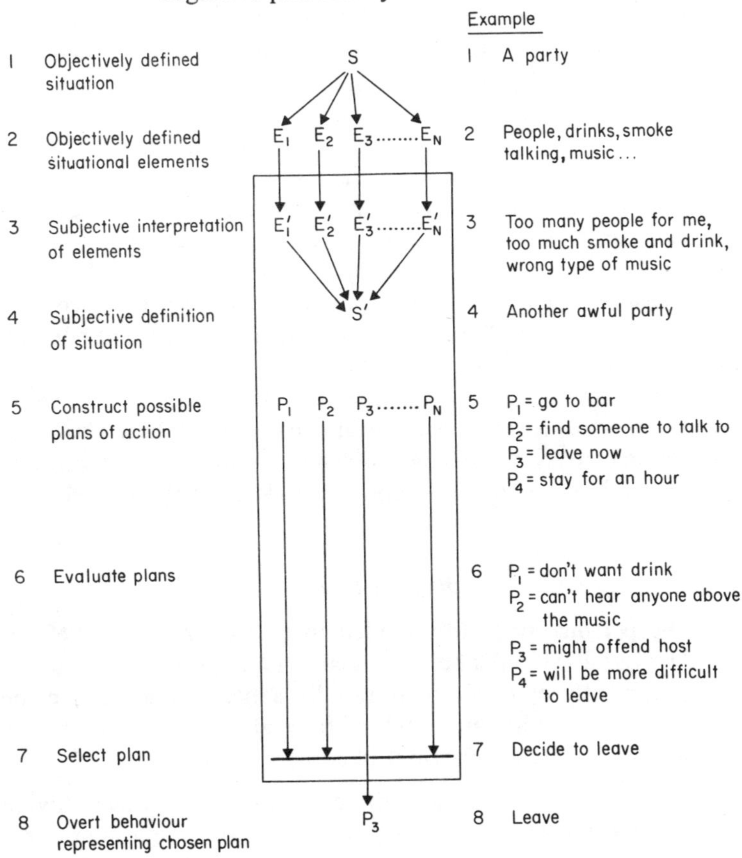

tion of behaviour. There are various ways in which brain differences may influence this process. Some might be that (a) males have less strongly lateralised brains, better arranged for parallel, spatial processing, whereas women are more attuned to sequential, verbal processing, so that males will attend more to visual, non-verbal cues in the situation while women attend more to verbal elements (Buffery, 1976), (b) individuals in a higher state of cortical arousal (e.g. introverts) will be able to attend to fewer situational elements given better concentration and narrower cue utilisation than individuals in a low state of arousal whose cortex is functioning less efficiently, (c) individuals in whom there is a high level of activity in a limbic-reticular or corticolimbic loop (e.g. neurotics) will be orientated more towards the affectively toned elements in a situation and tend to interpret stimulus elements in a more affectively toned manner than will the individual with low activity in these systems, (d) individuals in whom cortical, associative processing is impaired, such as when the cortex is lesioned, will show changes in the manner of interpreting elements, and, more specifically, will be forced to attend to fewer elements to reduce the processing load. This change would therefore be in the introverted direction, contrary to Eysenck's (1967) theories concerning the generally extraverting effects of drain damage. A reduction in the range of stimulus elements attended to may also cause a certain rigidity in behaviour since if a small number of elements is consistently attended to, there is a greater chance that any two given situations will be evaluated, and hence responded to, identically. If cortical damage is extreme it will severely reduce the individual's ability to adapt and respond flexibly to circumstances and will be one reason for the known relationship between cortical damage and psychiatric disability (Lishman, 1968; Hackney and Taylor, 1976), (e) individuals who have suffered lesions that interrupt the flow of information between cortex and limbic systems (e.g. cingulectomies, amygdalectomies and orbital undercuts) will pay less attention to the affective elements of situations and interpret situational elements in a less affectively toned manner. This is functionally equivalent to a reduction in neuroticism, and can be noted in frontal cases who talk quite blandly about objectively distressing problems, and in, say, cingulectomy cases who show a reduction in emotional responsivity (Kelly et al. 1973; Mitchell-Heggs et al., 1976).

Construction of possible plans of action

This is the personality ability alluded to by Miller et al. (1960), and partly assessed by Luria's (1966) laboratory tasks that require the individual to run two plans concurrently or to alternate rapidly between plans, and evidenced, for example, in the frontal case's lack of foresight and perseverative tendencies. Miller and his colleagues phrase it like this:

> Popular speech recognises differences in values by such sayings as 'One man's meat is another man's poison', 'There is no accounting for tastes,'

etc. We may even accuse each other of basic differences in our Images with such comments as, 'His ideas are weird', 'He doesn't speak our language', etc. But individuality is perhaps more often captured by such phrases as, 'John would have handled it differently', 'Bill would have done it like this', 'You never know what he will try next', 'They never give up', etc. These phrases relate to differences in the way people tackle a problem and carry it through.

Miller goes on the describe some of the obvious ways in which plan construction might differ: *source* (entirely from within or with the advice of others); *span* (encompassing the next few minutes, or hours, years or lifetimes); *detail* (from the smallest tactics to the broadest strategy); *flexibility* (the ability to interrupt and change easily between plans); *speed* (of construction) and so on.

When it comes to the neuropsychological basis of plan construction, Miller et al. are refreshingly blunt 'the authors are not sure where or how the brain might generate Plans'. But they do suggest that the primary construction areas will be in the posterior association cortex (i.e. temporal, occipital and parietal lobe cortex), although actual plan execution will be undertaken by the frontal cortex. This is a sufficiently clear statement to predict that cortical lesions will influence personality partly by reducing the individual's ability to create rapidly a series of possible plans of behaviour in a situation. The reduction in planning capacity may take the form of limiting the numbers of alternative plans constructed, by slowing the process, by reducing their internal detail, or in some as yet unpredicted manner. It can also be hypothesised that if the cortex undertakes plan construction in the absence of proper connectivity with the limbic system, that plans will be less affect-dominated and lead, for example, to less avoidance behaviour in previously high anxiety or high neurotic individuals.

Plan selection

Given that a series of possible plans has been generated, the next step is for the individual to select between them. This can be achieved by mentally running through a plan and assigning some value dependent on the desirability of the anticipated outcomes. Plan values are compared and the most attractive, or least objectionable, selected. Again, the intactness of the cortex would seem crucial for this task, that embodies the flavour of 'judgement' and 'foresight'. The inability to rehearse plan outcome properly must be expected to relate to the impulsive, ill-considered, inappropriate and maladaptive behaviours often exhibited by brain-damaged individuals.

Overall, we can see that a new approach to personality assessment leads us towards the measurement of certain cognitive abilities or person characteristics that may well have a basis in organic brain processing. Obviously a whole new range of assessment techniques has to be developed — to measure subjective

Fig. 8.2 A compilation of current neuropsychological models of personality, indicating the main places where the effects of lesions are evaluated

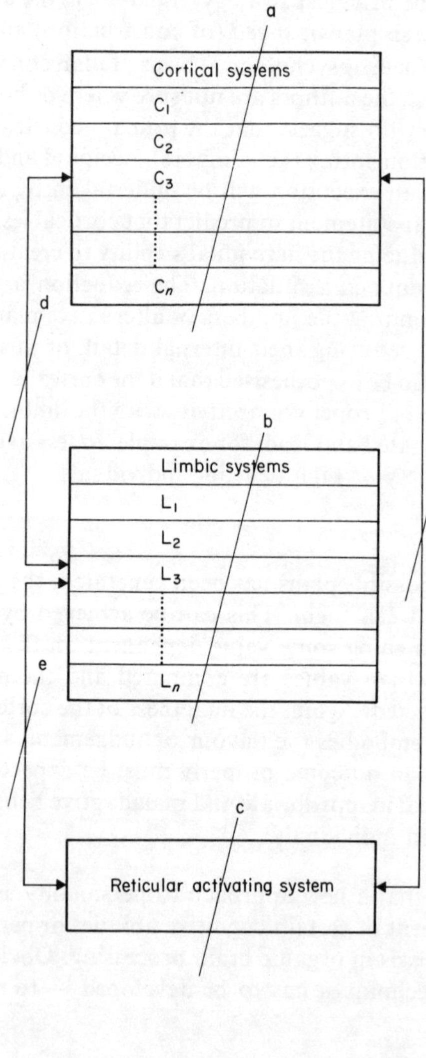

assessments of situations, the variety of plans constructed, the ability to predict plan outcome, and so on — but to the enterprising researcher this is the red meat of investigation.

A summary of actual and potential brain-personality relationships

Having discussed measurement issues, and pencilled in some new lines of research into brain-personality relationships through using different approaches to the assessment of emotions and personality, an attempt to summarise the whole area is in order.

The first point to make is that there is no one neuropsychological model of personality, and there can never be, because personality is such an inclusive term, implicating many processes, states and mechanisms, each of which may lay claim to its own neuropsychological theory. However, Fig. 8.2 goes some way towards representing the overall field. Research has been directed towards establishing the role of cortical, limbic and reticular systems in personality, and also the role of the connecting fibres between the three systems, that are viewed as loops or systems in their own right. One way of giving an overview of the area is to consider the effects, both actual and predicted, of lesions to the various aspects of this model, the lesions having been labelled a to f in the figure. Since details have been discussed in earlier chapters, only a brief concluding statement will be made concerning each.

(a) Cortical lesions

We know that a general intactness of the cortex is required or personality will tend to disintegrate in ways predisposing the individual to psychiatric illness, and we know that the left v. right distinction may be relevant to the precise type of psychiatric disability. Further, we know that various parts of the cortex may be especially relevant to particular aspects of personality in the way that temporal cortex has an association with aggression control; the orbital frontal cortex and cingulate gyrus have a role in the reception of mood states; and the prefrontal regions and remainder of the frontal lobes help generally to organise actions. In addition, we know that certain nuclear sites exist on the cortex to interpret sensory stimuli in all the modalities, but the relation between damage to these nuclear sites and personality is not known. Further research needs to concentrate on the role of the cortex in the integration of affective information into action, its role in the interpretation of situations (interpretations that will eventually guide behaviour), and its role in the construction of plans for behaviour.

(b) *Limbic lesions*

We know that there are many limbic circuits to consider, and many specific nuclear sites, which when stimulated or ablated may disrupt drive orientated and affective behaviour. We know, for example, that lesions to Papez's circuit can dampen behaviour intensity and inhibit negative emotional experience, and that hypothalamic lesions affect sex drive. Future research will depend on the delineation of other relevant circuits, such as described by Gray regarding the role of the hippocampus in extraversion; on more subtle measurement of affectively tinged performance; and on how the cortex copes with faulty or distorted limbic outpourings.

(c) *Reticular systems*

This system contains the major activating system for both cortex and limbic systems, and when lesioned can cause major fluctuations and shifts in arousal level. We know that drugs which dampen RAS activity tend to produce extraverted behaviour. Further exploration is required into the relationship of arousal to redundancy in processing, the relative balance of excitatory and inhibitory potentials considered separately, facets of discontinuous processing, the perception of situational determinants of behaviour, and to plan construction and evaluation.

(d) *Corticolimbic loop*

This helps towards exciting limbic circuits through psychic rather than visceral events. We know their lesioning reduces the experience of certain affective states. The disconnection of cortical from limbic circuits raises problems of how this influences normal mood and affective processing, and how the disconnection may alter planning and evaluative activities. This circuit is important in the maintenance of neuroticism. There are various corticolimbic connections each of which needs separate investigation, such as the difference between lesions to the frontal-limbic fibres and lesions to temporal-limbic fibres.

(e) Limbic-reticular loop

The limbic-reticular loop has been described by Eysenck as relevant to neuroticism, which it may well be. However, description and delineation is needed for the personality and behaviour differences between an individual with a limbic system activated from both cortical and reticular sources and an individual whose limbic system is activated solely from cortical sources. Gray has described one particular limbic-reticular loop that may be relevant to extraversion as well as neuroticism.

(f) Corticoreticular loop

Again, described by Eysenck as relevant to extraversion, which it may well be. It is clear from Fig. 8.2 that if an individual suffers a lesion at f then he or she will be left with an under-aroused cortex but normally activated limbic system, which would predict a predominance in cognition of limbic events and a concomitant increase in neurotic features. This possible state, another form of disconnection syndrome, needs investigation, as does the various impact of lesions to the different corticoreticular connections.

References

Allport, D.A. (1968). 'Phenomenal Simultaneity and the Perceptual Moment Hypothesis', *Brit. J. Psychol., 59*, 395-406.

Aman, M.G. (1978). 'Drugs, learning and the psychotherapics' in J.S. Werry (ed.), *Pediatric Psychopharmacology: the use of behaviour modifying drugs in children*, Brunner Mazel, New York.

Amsel, A. (1962). 'Frustrative Nonreward in Partial Reinforcement and Discrimination Learning: Some Recent History and a Theoretical Extension', *Psychol. Rev., 69*, 306-28.

Anderson, A.L. and Hanvik, L.J. (1950). 'The Psychometric Localization of Brain Lesions: the Differential Effect of Frontal and Parietal Lesions on MMPI Profiles', *J. clin. Psychol., 6*, 177-80.

Andrieux, C. (1955). 'Contribution a l'Etude des Differences entre Hommes et Femmes dans la Perception spatiale', *L'Annee Psychol., 55*, 41-60.

Andy, O.J. and Jurko, M.E. (1972a). 'Hyperresponsive syndrome' in E. Hitchcock, L. Laitinen and K. Vaernet (eds.), *Psychosurgery*, Charles C. Thomas, Springfield, Illinois.

Andy, O.J. and Jurko, M.F. (1972b). 'Thalamotomy for hyperresponsiveness syndrome: lesions in the centermedianum and intralaminar nuclei' in E. Hitchcock, L. Laitinen and K. Vaernet (eds.), *Psychosurgery*, Charles C. Thomas, Springfield, Illinois.

Argyle, M. (1969). *Social Interaction*, Methuen, London.

Bailey, H.R., Dowling, J.L. and Davies, E. (1977). 'Cingulotractotomy and related procedures for severe depressive illness', in W.H. Sweet, S. Obrador and J.G. Martin-Rodriguez (eds.), *Neurosurgical treatment in Psychiatry, Pain and epilepsy*, University Park Press, Baltimore.

Bakan, P., Belton, J.A. and Toth J.C. (1963). 'Extraversion-introversion and decrement in an auditory vigilance task in D.N. Buckner and J.T. McGarath (eds.), *Vigilance: A Symposium*, McGraw-Hill, New York.

Balasubramaniam, V., Ramanujam, P.B., Kanaka, T.S. and Ramanurthi, B. (1972). 'Stereotaxic surgery for behaviour disorders' in E. Hitchcock, L. Laitinen and K. Vaernet (eds.), *Psychosurgery*, Charles C. Thomas, Springfield, Illinois.

Ballantine, H.T. Jr, Cassidy, W., Flanagan, N.B. and Marino, E.R. (1967). 'Stereotaxic Anterior Cingulotomy for Neuropsychiatric Illness and Intractable Pain', *J. Neurosurg., 26*, 488-95.

Ballantine, H.T. Jr, Cassidy, W.C., Brodenr, J. and Giriunas, I. (1972). 'Frontal cingulotomy for mood disturbance' in E. Hitchcock, L. Laitinen and K.

Vaernet (eds.), *Psychosurgery*, Charles C. Thomas, Springfield, Illinois.
036Barkley, R.A. (1977). 'A Review of Stimulant Drug Research with Hyperactive Children', *J. child Psychol. and Psychiat.*, *18*, 137-65.

Bartenwerfer, H. (1957). 'Uber die Answirkungen einforuniger Arbeitsvorgange', *Sitzungberichte der Ges. z. Bef. de. ges. Naturwiss. zur Marburg.*, *80*, 1-70.

Bender, M.B. (1952). *Disorders in Perception*, Charles C. Thomas, Springfield, Illinois.

Bennett, D.H. (1956). 'Perception of the Upright in Relation to the Body Image', *J. ment. Sci.*, *102*, 487-506.

Bennett-Levy, J. (1978). 'Subjective memory,' unpublished M.Phil. thesis, University of London.

Bhatia, R. and Kollevold, T. (1976). 'A Follow-up Study of 91 Patients Operated on for Focal Epilepsy', *Epilepsia*, *17*, 61-6.

Blakemore, C.B. (1967). 'Personality and brain damage' in H.J. Eysenck (ed.), *Biological Basis of Behaviour*, Charles C. Thomas, Springfield, Illinois.

Blakemore, C.B. (1969). 'Psychological effects of temporal lobe lesions in man' in R.N. Herrington (ed.), '*Current Problems in Neuropsychiatry*', *Brit. J. Psychiatry.*, Special Publication no. 4.

Broadbent, D.E. (1956). 'Inhibition and Extraversion', *Q. Bull. Brit. Psychol. Soc.*, *29*, 13.

Broager, B. and Olesen, K. (1972). 'Psychosurgery in sixty-three cases of open cingulectomy and fourteen cases of bifrontal prehypothalmic cryolesion' in E. Hitchcock, L. Laitinen, and K. Vaernet (eds.), *Psychosurgery*, Charles C. Thomas, Springfield, Illinois.

Buffery, A.W.H. (1975). 'Sex differences in the neuropsychological development of verbal and spatial skills', paper presented to NATO conference, 'The neuropsychology of learning disorders: theoretical approaches', Korsor, Denmark.

Buffery, A.W.H. (1976). 'Sex differences in the neuropschological development of verbal and spatial skills', in R. Knights and D.J. Bakker (eds.), *The Neuropsychology of Learning Disorders: Theoretical Approaches*, University Park Press.

Buffery, A.W.H. (1977). 'Clinical neuropsychology: A review and preview' in S.J. Rachman (ed.), *Advances in Medical Psychology*, Pergammon Press, Oxford.

Buffery, A.W.H. and Gray, J.A. (1972). 'Sex differences in the development of spatial and linguistic skills' in C. Ounsted and D.C. Taylor (eds.), *Gender Differences: Their ontogeny and significance*, Churchill-Livingstone, London.

Butter, H. and Lapierre, Y. (1974). 'The effect of methylphenidate on sensory perception and integration in hyperactive children', *Int. Pharmacopsy-*

chiat., *9*, 235-44.

Butter, H. and Lapierre, Y. (1975). 'The Effect of Methylphenidate on Sensory Perception in Varying Degrees of Hyperkinetic Behaviour', *Dis. nerv. System.*, *36*, 286-8.

Butters, N. and Rosvold, H.E. (1968). 'Effect of Caundate and Septal Nuclei Lesions on Resistance to Extinction and Delayed Alternation', *J. comp. physiol. Psychol.*, *65*, 397-403.

Campbell, S., Douglas, V. and Morgenstern, G. (1971). 'Cognitive Styles in Hyperactive Children and the Effect of Methylphenidate', *J. child Psychol. Psychiat.*, *12*, 55-67.

Cantwell, D.P. and Carlson, G.A. (1978). 'Stimulants in J.S. Werry (ed.), *Pediatric Psychopharmacology: the use of behaviour modifying drugs in children*, Brunner Mazel, New York.

Choppy, M., Zimbacca, N. and Le Beau, J. (1973). 'Psychological changes after selective frontal surgery (especially cingulotomy) and after stereotactic surgery of the basal ganglia' in L.V. Laitinen and K.E. Livingston (eds), *Surgical Approaches in Psychiatry*, Medical and Technical Publishing, Lancester.

Claridge, G.S. (1956). *Factors Affecting the Motivation and Performance of Imbeciles',* PhD thesis, University of London.

Claridge, G.S. (1960). 'The excitation-inhibition balance in neurotics' in H.J. Eysenck (ed.), *Experiments in Personality*, *2*, Praeger, New York.

Cohen, N., Douglas, V. and Morgenstern, G. (1971). 'The Effect of Methylphenidate on Attentive Behaviour and Autonomic Activity in Hyperactive Children', *Psychopharmacologia*, *22*, 282-94.

Conners, C., Eisenberg, L. and Sharpe, L. (1964). 'Effects of Methylphenidate (Ritalin) on Paired Associate Learning and Porteus Maze Performance in Emotionally Disturbed Children', *J. consult. Psychol.*, *28*, 14-22.

Conners, C.K. (1972). 'Pharmacotherapy of psychopathy in children' in H. Quay and J. Werry (eds), *Psychopathological Disorders Of Childhood*, Wiley, New York.

Corbett, J.A. (1977). 'Tics and Tourette's syndrome' in M. Rutter and L. Hersov (eds), *Child Psychiatry: Modern Approaches*, Blackwell, Oxford.

Corcoran, D.W.J. (1964). 'Personality and the Inverted-U Relation', *Brit. J. Psychol.*, *56*, 267-74.

Costello, C.G. and Eysenck, H.J. (1966). 'Persistence, Personality and Motivation', *Percept. Mot. Skills*, *12*, 169-170.

Davis, D.R. (1946). 'Neurotic Disposition and the Disorganization Observed in Experiments with the Cambridge Cockpit', *J. Neurol. Neurosurg. J. Psychiat.*, *9*, 119-24.

Davis, D.R. (1968). *Pilot effort — some Laboratory Experiments*, HMSO, London.

Davis, D.R. (1949). 'The Disorder of Skill Responsible for Accidents', *Q. J. exp.*

Psychol., *1*, 136-42.

Dewson, J.H., Noble, K.W. and Pribram, K.H. (1966). 'Cortico-influence and Cochlear Nucleus of the Cat: Some Effects of Ablation of Insular-Temporal Cortex', *Brain Res.*, *62*, 123-24.

Dieckmann, G. and Hassler, R. (1977). 'Treatment of sexual violence by stereotactic hypothalamotomy, in W.H. Sweet, S. Obrador and J.G. Martin-Rodriguez (eds) *Neurosurgical treatment in Psychiatry, Pain, and Epilepsy*-,University Park Press, Baltimore.

Dikman, S.S. and Reitan, R.M. (1974). 'MMPI correlates of localized cerebral lesions', *Perc. Mot. Skills*, *39*, 831-40.

Dixon, N.F. (1971). *Subliminal Perception: the Nature of a Controversy*, McGraw-Hill, London.

Doehring, D.G. and Reitan, R.M. (1960) MMPI performance of aphasic and nonaphasic brain-damaged patients, *J. clin. Psychol.*, *16*, 307-9.

Douglas, V. (1974). 'Differences between normal and hyperkinetic children' in C. Conners (ed.), *Clinical Use of Stimulant Drugs in Children*, Elsevier, Amsterdam.

Drewe, E.A. (1973). 'An experimental investigation of deficits found following lesions in the frontal lobes'. unpublished PhD thesis, University of London.

Dunstone, J.J., Dzendolot, G. and Henckeruth, O. (1964). 'Effect of some Personality Variables on Electrical Vestibular Stimulation', *Percept. Mot. Skills.*, *18*, 689-95.

Endler, N.S. and Magnusson, D. (1976). 'Towards an Interactional Psychology of Personality', *Psychol. Bull.*, *83*, 956-74.

Eysenck, H.J. (1957). *Dynamics of Anxiety and Hysteria*, Routledge and Kegan Paul, London.

Eysenck, H.J. (1964). 'Involuntary Rest Pauses in Tapping as a Function of Drive and Personality', *Perc. Mot. Skills*, *18*, 173-4.

Eysenck, H.J. (1965). 'Extraversion and the Acquisition of Eyeblink and GSR Conditioned Responses', *Psych. Bull.*, *63*, 258-70.

Eysenck, H.J. (1967). *The Biological Basis of Personality*, Charles C. Thomas, Springfield, Illinois.

Eysenck, H.J. (1971). 'Human typology, higher nervous activity and factor analysis' in V.D. Nebylitsyn T.A. and J.A. Gray (eds), *Biological Bases of Individual Behaviour*, Academic Press, London.

Eysenck, H.J. (ed.) 1979). *A Model of Personality*, in press.

Eysenck, H.J. and Levey, A. (1967). 'Konditionierung, Introversion-Extraversion und die Starke des Nervensystems' *Zeitschift fur Psychologie*, *174*, 96-106.

Eysenck, H.J. and Eysenck, S.B.G. (1976). *Psychoticism as a Dimension of Personality*, Hodder and Stoughton, London.

Eysenck, H.J. and Frith, C.D. (1977). *Reminiscence, Motivation and Personality*, Plenum Press, New York.

Falconer, M.A. (1973). 'Reversibility by Temporal-lobe Resection of the Behavioural Abnormalities of Temporal-lobe Epilepsy, *New. Eng. J. Med.*, 289, 451-55.

Falconer, M.A., Hill, D., Meyer, A., Mitchell, W. and Pond, D.A. (1955). 'Treatment of Temporal Lobe Epilepsy by Temporal Lobectomy. A Survey of Findings and Results', *Lancet*, *Vol. i*, 827-35.

Flor-Henry, P. (1969). 'Psychosis and Temporal Lobe Epilepsy. A Controlled Investigation', *Epilepsia, 10*, 363-88.

Flor-Henry, P. (1969). 'Schizophrenia-like Reactions and Affective Psychoses Associated with Temporal Lobe Epilepsy: Etiological Factors', *Am. J. Psychiat., 126*, 148-52.

Flor-Henry, P. (1973). 'Psychiatric syndromes considered as manifestations of lateralized temporal-limbic dysfunction' in L.V. Laitinen and K.E. Livingston (eds), *Surgical Approaches in Psychiatry*, Medical and Technical Publishing, Lancaster.

Franks, C.M. (1954). *An Experimental Study of Conditioning as Related to Mental Abnormality*, PhD thesis, University of London.

Franks, C.M. (1956). 'Recidivism, Psychopathy and Personality', *Brit. J. Delinq.*, *6*, 192-201.

Franks, C.M. (1956). 'Conditioning and Personality: A Study of Normal and Neurotic Subjects', *J. abn. Soc. Psychol.*, *52*, 143-50.

Franks, C.M. (1957). 'Personality Factors and the Rate of Conditioning', *Brit. J. Psychol.*, *48*, 119-26.

Franks, C.M. (1963). 'Ocular Movements and Spontaneous Blink Rate as Functions of Personality', *Percept. Mot. Skills*, *16*, 178.

Franks, C.M. and Trouton, D.S. (1957). 'The effects of stimulant and depressant drugs upon conditioning in man' reported in H.J. Eysenck, *Dynamics of Anxiety and Hysteria*, Routledge and Kegan Paul, London.

Freeman, W. (1973). 'Sexual Behaviour and Fertility after Frontal Lobectomy', *Biol. Psychiat.*, *6*, 97-104.

Friedman, R., Dale, E. and Wagner, J. (1973). 'A Long-term Comparison of Two Treatment Regimens for Minimal Brain Dysfunction', *Clin. Pediatrics*, *12*, 666-71.

Fulton, J.F. (1951). *Frontal Lobotomy and Affective Behaviour. A Neurophysiological Analysis*, Norton, New York.

Furneaux, D. (1955). *Manual of Nufferno Speed Tests*, National Foundation Educational Research, 18.

Garfinkel, B., Webster, C. and Sloman, L. (1978). 'Methylphenidate and Caffeine in the Treatment of Children with Minimal Brain Dysfunction', *Am. J. Psychiat.*, *132*, 723-28.

Garner, W.R. (1962). *Uncertainty and Structure as Psychological Concepts*, Wiley, New York.

Gebhart, R. (1966). Dusseldorf, Psychol. Inst; unpublished work.

Geschwind, N. (1965). 'Disconnexion Syndromes in Animals and Man', *Brain, 88*, 237-94.

Gittelman-Klein, R. and Klein, D. (1976). 'Methylphenidate Effects in Learning Disabilities: Psychometric Changes', *Arch. gen. Psychiat.*, *33*, 655-64.

Goldstone, S. (1955). 'Flicker Fusion Measurements and Anxiety Level', *J. exp. Psychol.*, *49*, 200-202.

Goodglass, H. and Blumstein, S. (1973). *Psycholinguistics and Aphasia*, John Hopkins Press, Baltimore.

Graham, P. and Rutter, M. (1968). 'Organic Brain Dysfunction and Child Psychiatric Disorder', *Brit. med. J., 3*, 695-700.

Gray, J.A. (1964). *Pavlov's Typology*, Pergammon, Oxford.

Gray, J.A. (1967). 'Strength of the Nervous System, Introversion, Conditionability and Arousal', *Behav. Res. Ther.*, *5*, 151-69.

Gray, J.A. and Smith, P.T. (1969). 'An arousal-decision model for partial reinforcement and discrimination learning' in R. Gilbert and N.S. Sutherland (eds), *Animal Discrimination Learning*, Academic Press, London.

Gray, J.A. (1970). 'The Psycho-physiological Basis of Introversion-Extraversion', *Behav. Res. Ther.*, *8*, 249-66.

Gray, J.A. (1972). 'The psychophysiological nature of introversion-extraversion: a modification of Eysenck's theory' in V.D. Nebylitsyn and J.A. Gray (eds), *Biological Bases of Individual Behaviour*, Academic Press, London.

Grossman, S.P. (1967). *A Textbook of Physiological Psychology*, John Wiley and Sons, New York.

Gupta, B.S. (1974). 'Stimulant and depressant drugs on kinaesthetic figural after effects', *Psychophamacologia (Berl.) 36*, 275-87.

Gupta, B.S. and Kaur, S. (1978). 'The Effects of Dextroamphetamine on Kinesthetic Figural after Effects', *Psychopharmacology, 56*, 199-204.

Gupta, B.S. and Singh, S.D. (1971). 'The Effect of Extraversion, Neuroticism and a Depressant Drug on Verbal Conditioning', *Ind. J. exp. Psychol.*, *5*, 15-17.

Hackney, A. and Taylor, D.C. (1976). 'A Teachers' Questionnaire Description of Epileptic Children', *Epileptic*, *17*, 275-81.

Harter, M.R. (1967). 'Excitability Cycles and Cortical Scanning. A Review of Two Hypotheses of Central Intermittency in Perception', *Psychol. Bull.*, *68*, 47-58.

Haslam, D.R. (1966). 'Individual differences in pain threshold and the concept of arousal', unpublished PhD thesis, Bristol University.

Hecaen, H. (1964). 'Mental symptoms associated with tumors of the frontal lobe' in J.M. Warren and K. Akert (eds), *The Frontal Granular Cortex and Behaviour*, McGraw-Hill, New York.

Hetherington, R.E., Haden, P. and Craig, W.J. (1972). 'Neurosurgery in affective disorder: criteria for selection of patients' in E. Hitchcock, L. Laitinen and K. Vaernet (eds), *Psychosurgery*, Charles C. Thomas, Springfield, Illinois.

Hill, D., Pond, D.A., Mitchell, W. and Falconer, M.A. (1957). 'Personality Changes following Temporal Lobectomy for Epilepsy', *J. ment. Sci., 103*, 18-27.

Hitchcock, E., Laitinen, L. and Vaernet, K. (eds). (1972), *Psychosurgery*, Charles C. Thomas, Springfield, Illinois.

Hitchcock, E.R., Ashcroft, G.W., Cairns, W.M. and Murray, L.G. (1972). 'Pre-operative and post-operative assessment and management of psychosurgical patients' in E. Hitchcock, L. Laitinen and K. Vaernet (eds), *Psychosurgery*, Charles C. Thomas, Springfield, Illinois.

Hitchcock, E.R., Ashcroft, G.W., Cairns, W.M. and Murray, L.G. (1973). 'Observations on the development of an assessment scheme for amygdalotomy' (L.V. Laitinen and K.E. Livingston (eds), *Surgical Approaches in Psychiatry*, Medical and Technical Publishing, Lancaster.

Hoffman, S., Engelhardt, D., Margolis, R., Polizos, P., Waizer, J. and Rosenfeld, R. (1974). 'Response to Methylphenidate in Low Socioeconomic Hyperactive Children', *Arch. gen. Psychiat., 30*, 354-9.

Hogan, M.J. (1968). 'Influence of Motivation on Reactive Inhibition in Extraversion-Introversion', *Perc. Mot. Skills., 22*, 187-92.

Hogan, R., De Soto, C. and Solano, C. (1977). 'Traits, Tests and Personality Research', *Amer. Psychol., 32*, 255-64.

Holland, H.C. (1963). '"Visual Masking" and the effects of stimulant and depressant drugs' in H.J. Eysenck (ed.), *Experiments with Drugs*, Pergammon, New York.

Holland, H.C. (1965). *The Spiral After-effect*, Pergammon, London.

Homskaya, E.D. (1973). 'The Human Frontal Lobes and their Role in the Organisation of Activity', *Acta neurobiol. Experimentalis, 33*, 509-22.

Isaacson, R.L. (1974). *The Limbic System*, Plenum Press, New York.

Janssen, R.H.C., Mattie, H., Plooij-Van Gorsel, P.C. and Werre, P.F. (1978). 'The Effects of a Depressant and a Stimulant Drug on the Contingent Negative Variation', *Biol. Psychol., 6*, 209-18.

Jawanda, J.S. (1966). 'Age, sex and personality variables in verbal conditioning and its modification by drugs', unpublished PhD thesis, Punjab University.

Jensen, A. (1964). *Individual Differences in Learning: Interference Factor*, US Department of Health, Education and Welfare, Project Report 1867.

Jones, B.E., Ayres, J.J.B., Flanary, H.C. and Clements, T.H. (1965). 'Effects of Morphine and Pentobarbital on Conditioned Electrodermal Responses and Basal Conductance in Man', *Psychopharmacologia, 7*, 159-74.

Kamano, D.K., Martin, L.K. and Powell, B.J. (1966). 'Avoidance Response Acquisition and Amobarbital Dosage Levels', *Psychopharmacologia, 8*, 319-23.

Karp, S.A. (1963). 'Field Dependence and Overcoming Embeddedness', *J. con-*

sult. Psychol., *27*, 194-302.

Kelly, D. (1973). 'Stereotactic Limbic Leucotomy; a preliminary report on forty patients', *Brit. J. Psychiat.*, *123*, 141-8.

Kelly, D. (1973). 'Therapeutic Outcome in Limbic Leucotomy in Psychiatric Patients', *Psychiatria, Neurologia, Neurochirurgia, 76*, 353-63.

Kelly, D., Richardson, A. and Mitchell-Heggs, N. (1973). 'Stereotactic Limbic Leucotomy: Neurophysiological Aspects and Operative Technique, *Brit. J. Psychiat.*, *123*, 133-40.

Kelly, D.H.W., Walter, C.T.S. and Sargant, W. (1966). 'Modified Leucotomy Assessed by Forearm Blood flow and other Measurements', *Brit. J. Psychiat.*, *112*, 871-81.

Kelvin, P. (1969). *The Bases of Social Behaviour*, Holt, Rinehart and Winston, London.

Kristofferson, A.B. (1967). 'Successive Discriminations as a Two-state Quantal Process', *Science*, *158*, 1337.

Krugman, H.E. (1947). 'Flicker Fusion Frequency as a Function of Anxiety Reaction: An Exploratory Study', *Psychosom. Med.*, *9*, 269-72.

Laitinen, L.V. and Livingston, K.E. (1973). *Surgical Approaches to Psychiatry*, Medical and Technical Publishing, Lancaster.

Laitinen, L.V. and Vilkki, J. (1972). 'Stereotaxic central anterior cingulotomy in some psycholgocial disorders,' in E. Hitchcock, L. Laitinen and K. Vaernet (eds), *Psychosurgery*, Charles C. Thomas, Springfield, Illinois.

Laitiner, L.V. and Vilkki, J. (1973). 'Observations on the transcallosal emotional connections' in L.V. Laitinen and K.E. Livingstone (eds), *Surgical Approaches in Psychiatry*, Medical and Technical Publishing, Lancaster.

Le Beau, J. (1954). *Psychochirurgie et Fonctions mentales*, Masson, Paris.

Levinson, F. and Meyer, V. (1965). 'Personality Changes in Relation to Psychiatric States following Orbital Cortex Undercutting', *Brit. J. Psychiat.*, *111*, 207-18.

Lishman, W.A. (1968). 'Brain Damage in Relation to Psychiatric Disability after Head Injury', *Brit. J. Psychiat.*, *114*, 373-410.

Livingston, K.E. and Escobar, A. (1972). 'The continuing evolution of the limbic system concept' in E. Hitchcock, L. Laitinen and K. Vaernet (eds), *Psychosurgery*, Charles C. Thomas, Springfield, Illinois.

Louks, J., Calsyn, D. and Lindsay, F. (1976). 'Personality Dysfunction and Lateralized Deficits in Cerebral Functions as Measured by the MMPI and Reitan-Halstead Battery, *Perc. Mot. Skills*, *43*, 655.

Luria, A.R. (1966). *Higher Cortical Functions in Man*, Tavistock Publications, London.

Lynn, R. (1960). 'Extraversion, Reminiscence and Satiation Effects', *Brit. J. Psychol.*, *51*, 319-24.

Lynn, R. and Eysenck, H.J. (1961). 'Tolerance for Pain, Extraversion and Neuroticism', *Perc. Mot. Skills, 12*, 161-2.

Mackay, D.M. (1953). 'Some Experiments on the Perception of Patterns Modulated by the Alpha Frequency', *EEG, 5*, 559-62.

Mackworth, H. (1948). 'Researches in the measurement of human performance', MRC Special Report no. 268, HMSO, London.

MacLean, P.D. and Delgado. J.M.R. (1963). 'Electrical and Chemical Stimulation of Fronto-Temporal Portion of Limbic System in the Working Animal', *Electroenceph. clin. Neurophysiol., 5*, 91-100.

Malmo, R.B. (1959). 'Activation: A Neurophysiological Dimension', *Psychol. Rev., 66*, 367-86.

Malmo, R.B. and Amsel, A. (1948). 'Anxiety Produced Interference in Serial Rote Learning with Observations on Rote Learning after Partial Frontal Lobectomy', *J. exp. Psychol., 38*, 440-54.

Mangan, G.L. (1974). 'Personality and Conditioning: Some Personality, Cognitive and Psycho-physiological Parameters of Classical Appetitive (Sexual) GSR Conditioning', *Pav. J. biol. Sci., 9*, 125-35.

Mark, V.H., Sweet, W.H. and Ervin, F.R. (1972), 'The effect of amygdelotomy on violent behaviour in patients with temporal lobe epilepsy' in E. Hitchcock, L. Laitinen and K. Vaernet (eds), *Psychosurgery*, Charles C. Thomas, Springfield, Illinois.

Marks, I.M., Birley, J.L.T. and Gelder, M.G. (1966). 'Modified Leucotomy in Severe Agoraphobia: A Controlled Serial Inquiry', *Brit. J. Psychiat., 112*, 757-69.

Martin, M. and Urban, Ya. (1966). 'An Electroencephalographic Investigation of Individual Differences in the Processes of Conditioning', *Proc. XVIII int. Cong. exp. Psychol.,* Moscow.

McIntyre, M., Pritchard, P.B. and Lombroso, C.T. (1976). 'Left and Right Temporal Lobesepileptics: A Controlled Investigation of Some Psychological Differences', *Epilepsia, 17*, 377-86.

McManis, D.C., McCarthy, M. and Koval, R. (1978). 'Effects of a Stimulant Drug on Extraversion Level in Hyperactive Children', *Perc. Mot. Skills, 46*, 88-90.

Meier, M. (1969). 'The regional localisation hypothesis and personality changes associated with focal cerebral lesions and ablations' in J.N. Butcher (ed.), *MMPI research development and clinical applications*, McGraw-Hill, New York.

Meier, M.J. and French, L.A. (1965). 'Some Personality Correlates of Unilateral and Bilateral EEG Abnormalities in Psychomotor Epileptics', *J. clin. Psychol., 31*, 3-9.

Meyer A. and Beck E., (1954). *Prefrontal Leucotomy and Related Operations: Anatomical Aspects of Success and Failure*, Oliver and Boyd, Edinburgh.

Meyer, G., McElhaney, M., Martin, W. and McGraw, C.P. (1973). 'Stereotactic cingulotomy with results of acute stimulation and serial psychological testing' in Laitinen, L.V. and K.E. Livingston (eds), *Surgical Approaches in*

Psychiatry, Medical and Technical Publishing, Lancaster.
Miller, G.A., Galanter, E. and Pribram, K.H. (1960). *Plans and the Structure of Behaviour*, Holt, Rinehart, and Winston, London.
Miller, N.E. (1959). 'Liberalisation of basis S-R Concepts: Extensions to conflict behaviour, motivation and social learning' in S. Koch (ed.), *Psychology: A Study of Science*, McGraw-Hill, New York.
Mingrino, S. and Schergna, E. (1972). 'Stereotaxic anterior cingulotomy in the treatment of severe behaviour disorders' in E. Hitchcock, L. Laitinen and K. Vaernet (eds), *Psychosurgery*, Charles C. Thomas, Springfield, Illinois.
Mischel, W. (1968). *Personality and Assessment*, Wiley, New York.
Mischel, W. (1969). 'Continuity and Change in Personality', *Amer. Psychol.*, *24*, 1012-18.
Mischel, W. (1973). 'Towards a Cognitive Social Learning Reconceptualization of Personality', *Psychol. Rev.*, *80*, 252-83.
Mischel, W. (1977). 'On the Future of Personality Measurement', *Amer. Psychol.*, *32*, 246-54.
Mitchell-Heggs, N., Kelly, D. and Richardson, A. (1976). 'Stereotactic Limbic Leucotomy — A Follow-up at 16 Months', *Brit. J. Psychiat.*, *128*, 226-40.
Narabayashi, H., Nagao, T., Saito, T., Yoshida, M. and Nazahata, M. (1963). 'Stereotaxic Amygdalotomy for Behaviour Disorders', *Arch. Neurol.*, *9*, 1-16.
Narabayashi, H. and Shima, F. (1973). 'Which is the better target, the medial or lateral nuclei? (for behaviour problems and paroxysm in epileptics), in L.V. Laitinen and K.E. Livingston (eds), *Surgical Approaches in Psychiatry*, Medical and Technical Publishing, Lancaster.
Nauta, W.J.M. (1971). 'The Problem of the Frontal Lobe. A reinterpretation', *J. Psychiat. Res.*, *8*, 167-87.
Nebylitsyn, V.D. (1963). 'The Structure of the Fundamental Properties of the Nervous System', *Vopr. Psikhol*, *4*, 21-34.
Nebylitsyn, V.D. (1966). *Basic Properties of the Nervous System in Man*, G.L. Mangan (ed., English edition), Plenum Press, New York.
Nebylitsyn, V.D. and Gray, J.A. (eds) (1972). *Biological Bases of Individual Behaviour*, Academic Press, London.
Nebylitsyn, V.D., Rozhdestvenskaya, V.I. and Teplov, B.M. (1960). 'Concerning the Interrelation between Absolute Sensitivity and Strength of the Nervous System', *Q. J. exp. Psychol.*, *12*, 17-25.
Oatley, K. (1969). 'Judging the Order of Visual Stimuli', *Q. J. exp. Psychol.*, *21*, 172-80.
Obrador, S. (1972). 'Observations and reflections on psychosurgery at different levels' in E. Hitchcock, L. Laitinen and K. Vaernet (eds), *Psychosurgery*, Charles C. Thomas, Springfield, Illinois.
Ornstein, R.E. (1972). *The Psychology of Consciousness*, Penguin, Harmondsworth, Middlesex.

Papez, J.W. (1937). 'A Proposed Mechanism of Emotion', *Arch. Neurol. Psychiat.*, *38*, 725-43.

Passingham, R.E. (1970). 'The Neurological Basis of Introversion-Extraversion: Gray's Theory', *Behav. Res. Ther.*, *8*, 353-66.

Pavlov, I.P. (1928) *Lectures on Conditioned reflex* Translated and edited by W.H. Gantt, Vol. 1, International Publishers, New York,

Petri, A. (1942). *Personality and the Frontal Lobes*, Routledge and Kegan Paul, London.

Petrie, A. and Le Beau, J. (1953). 'The Psychological Effects of Selective Frontal Surgery including Cingulectomy', *Proc. Ve. Cong. Neurologique intern; Lisbonne*, *2*, 215.

Pippard, J. (1955). 'Personality Change after Rostral Leucotomy: A Comparison with Standard Prefrontal Leucotomy', *J. ment. Sci.*, *101*, 774-87.

Post, F., Linford Rees, W. and Schurr, P.H. (1968). 'An Evaluation of Bimedial Leucotomy', *Brit. J. Psychiatry*, *14*, 1223-46.

Pribram, K.H. (1968). 'Toward a neuropsychological theory of person' in K.H. Pribram (ed.), *The Study of Personality: An Interdisciplinary Approach*, Holt, Rinehart and Winston, New York.

Rapoport, J., Quinn, P. Bradbard, G., Riddle, D. and Brookes, E. (1974). 'Imipramine and Methylphenidate Treatment of Hyperactive Boys: A Double Blind Comparison, *Arch. gen. Psychiat.*, *30*, 789-93.

Rachman, S. and Hodgson, R. (1974). 'I. Synchrony and Desynchrony in Fear and avoidance', *Behav. Res. Ther.*, *12*, 311-18.

Riechard, C.C. and Elder, S.T. (1977). 'The Effects of Caffeine on Reaction Time in Hyperkinetic and Normal Children', *Amer. J. Psychiat.*, *134*, 144-8.

Richards, T.W. (1952). 'Personality of the Convulsive Patient in the Military Service', *Psychol. Monog.*, *16*, whole 346.

Roeder, F., Orthner, H. and Muller, D. (1972) 'The stereotaxic treatment of pedophilic homosexuality and other sexual deviations' in E. Hitchcock, L. Laitinen and K. Vaernet (eds), *Psychosurgery*, Charles C. Thomas, Springfield, Illinois.

Roberts, A.H. (1969). *Brain Damage in Boxers*, Pitman, London.

Rosenman, M.F. and Lucik T.W. (1970). 'A Failure to Replicate an Epilepsy Scale of the MMPI', *J. clin. Psychol.*, *26*, 372.

Rozhdestvenskaya, V.I. (1959). 'The strength of the nervous system as shown in the ability of nerve cells to endure protracted concentrated excitation' in J.A. Gray (ed.), *Pavlov's Typology*, Pergammon, Oxford.

Rutter, M. (1977). 'Brain Damage Syndromes in Childhood: Concepts and Findings *J. child Psychol. Psychiat.*, *18*, 1-21.

Rutter, M.A., Tizard, J. and Whitmore, K. (1970). *Education, Health and Behaviour*, Longmans, London.

Sano, K., Sekino, H. and Mayanagi, Y. (1972). 'Results of stimulation and destruction of the posterior hypothalamus in cases with violent, aggressive or restless behaviours' in E. Hitchcock, L. Laitinen and K. Vaernet (eds), *Psychosurgery*, Charles C. Thomas, Springfield, Illinois.

Satterfield, J. (1973). 'EEG Issues in Children with Minimal Brain Dysfunction', *Seminars in Psychiatry*, *5*, 35-46.

Satterfield, J. (1978). 'The hyper-active child syndrome: A precursor of adult psychopathy?' in R.D. Hare and D. Schalling (eds), *Psychopathic Behaviour: Approaches to Research*, Wiley, Chichester.

Satterfield, J., Cantwell, D., Lesser, L. and Podosin, R. (1972). 'Physiological Studies of the Hyperkinetic Child', *Amer. J. Psychiat.*, *128*, 102-8.

Satterfield, J., Cantwell, D. and Satterfield, B. (1974) 'Patho-physiology of the Hyperactive Child Syndrome', *Arch. gen. Psychiat.*, *31*, 839-44.

Satterfield, J. and Dawson, M. (1971). 'Electrodermal Correlates of Hyperactivity in Children', *Psychophysiology*, *8*, 191-7.

Savage, R.D. (1964). 'Electro-cerebral Activity, Extraversion and Neuroticism', *Brit. J. Psychiat.*, *110*, 98-100.

Seidel, U.P., Chadwick, O.F.D. and Rutter, M. (1975) 'Psychological Disorders in Crippled Children. A Comparative Study of Children with and without Brain Damage', *Dev. med. child Neurol.*, *17*, 563-73.

Semmes, J. (1968). 'Hemispheric Specialization: Possible Clues to Mechanisms', *Neuropsychologia*, *6*, 11-26.

Shaffer, D., Chadwick, O. and Rutter, M. (1975). 'Psychiatric outcome of localized head injury in children' in *Outcome of Severe damage to the central nervous system*, Elsevier, Amsterdam.

Shagass, C. (1954). 'The Sedation Threshold. A Method for Estimating Tension in Psychiatric patients, *Electroenceph. clin. Neurophysiol.*, *6*, 221-33.

Shagass, C. (1955). 'Anxiety, Depression, and the Photically Driven EEG', *A.M.A. Arch. Neurol. Psychiat.*, *74*, 3-10.

Shagass, C. (1956). 'Sedation Threshold: A Neurophysiological Tool for Psychosomatic Research', *Psychosom. Med.*, *18*, 410-19.

Shallice, T. (1964). 'The Detection of Chnage and the Perceptual Moment Hypothesis', *Brit. J. stat. Psychol.*, *17*, 113-35.

Skanthakumari, S.K. (1965). 'Personality Differences in the Rate of Forgetting', *J. ind. acad. appl. Psychol.*, *2*, 39-47.

Smith, J.S., Kiloh, L.G. and Boots, J.A. (1977) 'Prospective evaluation of prefrontal leucotomy: Results of 30 months follow-up', in W.H. Sweet, S. Obrador and J.G. Martin-Rodriguez (eds) *Neurosurgical treatment in Psychiatry, pain, and epilepsy*, University Park Press, Baltimore.

Smith, S.L. (1960). 'The effect of personality and drugs on auditory threshold when risk-taking factors are controlled' reported in H.J. Eysenck (1967), *Biological Basis of Personality*, Charles C. Thomas, Springfield, Illinois.

Spence, K.W. (1964). 'Anxiety (Drive) Level and Performance in Eyelid Conditioning', *Psych. Bull.*, *61*, 129-39.

Spielman, I.G.E. (1963). 'The relation between personality and the frequency and duration of involuntary rest pauses during named practice', unpublished PhD thesis, University of London.

Spinelli, D.N. and Pribram, K.H. (1966). 'Changes in Visual Recovery Functions Produced by Temporal Lobe Stimulation in Monkeys', *Electroenceph. clin. Neurophysiol., 20*, 44-49.

Spinelli, D.N. and Pribram, K.H. (1967). 'Changes in Visual Recovery Function and Unit Activity Produced by Frontal Cortex Stimulation', *EEG clin. Neurophysiol., 22*, 143-9.

Steinberg, H. and Summerfield, A. (1955). 'Effects of Nitrous Oxide on Learning and Retention', *Bull. Brit. Psychol. Soc., 6*, 6-7.

Stumpf, C. (1965). 'Drug Action on the Electrical Activity of the Hippocampus'. *Intern. Rev. Neurobiol., 8*, 77-138.

Surwillow, W.W. (1964). 'The Relation of Decision Time to Brain Wave Frequency and to Age', *EEG 16*, 510-14.

Tan, E., Marks, I.M. and Marset, P. (1971). 'Bimedial Leucotomy in Obsessive-Compulsive Neurosis: A Controlled Serial Inquiry', *Brit. J. Psychiat., 118*, 155-64.

Teplov, B.M. (1964). 'Problems in the study of general types of higher nervous activity in man and animals' in J.A. Gray (ed.), *Pavlov's Typology*, Pergammon Press, Oxford.

Teplov, B.M. (1964). *Problems of Individual Differences*, Moscow.

Tow, P.M. (1955). *Personality Changes following Frontal Leucotomy*, Oxford Medical Publications, London.

Tow, P.M. and Whitty, C.W.M. (1953). 'Personality Changes after Operations on the Cingulate Gyrus in Man', *J. Neurol. Neurosurg. Psychiat., 16*, 186-93.

Treadwell, G. (1956). *Motor Reminiscence and individual personality differences*, unpublished BA thesis, University of Belfast.

Ursin, H. (1960). 'The Temporal Lobe Substrate of Fear and Anger', *Acta. Psychiat. Neurol. Scand., 35*, 378-96.

Vaernet, K. and Madsen, A. (1970). 'Stereotaxic Amygdalotomy and Basofrontal Tractotomy in Psychotics with Aggressive Behaviour', *J. Neurol. Neurosurg. Psychiat., 33*, 858-67.

Venables, P.H. (1953). *A Study of Motor and Autonomic Responses to Experimentally Induced Stress in an Industrial Setting*, unpublished PhD thesis, University of London.

Venables, P.H. (1955). 'Change in Motor Response with Increase and Decrease in Task Difficulty in Normal Industrial and Psychiatric Patient Subjects', *Brit. J. Psychol., 46*, 101-10.

Venables, P.H. (1956). 'Some Findings on the Relationship between GSR and Motor Task Variables', *J. gen. Psychol., 55*, 199-202.

Vidor, M. (1951). 'Personality Changes following Prefrontal Leucotomy as Reflected by the MMPI and the Results of Psychometric Testing', *J. ment. Sci.*, *97*, 159-73.

Walsh, K.W. (1977). 'Neuropsychological aspects of modified leucotomy', in W.H. Sweet, S. Obrador and J.G. Martin-Rodriguez (eds), *Neurosurgical treatment in Psychiatry, pain, and epilepsy,* University Park Press, Baltimore.

Weil, J.L. (1974). *A Neurophysiological Model of Emotional and Intentional Behaviour*, Charles C. Thomas, Springfield, Illinois.

Weisen, A. (1965). 'Differential reinforcing effects of onset and offset of stimulation on the operant behaviour of normals neurotics and psychopaths', unpublished PhD thesis, University of Florida.

Weiss, G., Kruger, E., Danielson, U. and Elman, M. (1975). 'Effect of long-term Treatment of Hyperactive Children with Methylphenidate', *Can. med. Assoc. J., 123*, 159-65.

Weiss, G., Minde, K., Douglas, V., Werry, J. and Sykes, D. (1971). 'Comparison of the Effects of Chlorpromazine, Dextroamphetamine, and Methylphenidate on the Behaviour and Intellectual Functioning of Hyperactive children', *Can. med. Assoc. J.*, *104*, 20-25.

Werry, J.S. (ed.) (1978). *Pediatric Psychopharmacology: The Use of Behaviour Modifying Drugs in Children*, Brunner Mazel, New York.

Werry, J. and Aman, M. (1975). 'Methylphenidate and Haloperidol in Children. Effects on Attention, Memory and Activity', *Arch. gen. Psychiat.*, *32*, 790-5.

Wiggin, J.S. (1973). *Personality and Prediction: Principles of Personality Assessment*, Addison-Wesley, New York.

Willett, R. (1960). 'The effects of psychosurgical procedures on behaviour' in H.J. Eysenck (ed.), *Handbook of Abnormal Psychology*, Pitman, London.

Williams, H.L. (1952). 'The Development of a Candality Scale for the MMPI', *J. clin. Psychol.*, *8*, 293-7.

Winsberg, B.G. and Yepes, L.E. (1978) 'Antipsychotics (major tranquilizers, neuroleptics)' in J.S. Werry (ed.), *Pediatric Psychopharmacology: the use of behaviour modifying drugs in children*, Brunner Mazel, New York.

Witelson, S.F. and Paillie, W. (1973). 'Left Hemisphere Specialisation for Language in the Newborn: Neuroanatomical Evidence of Asymmetry', *Brain*, *96*, 641-6.

Witkin, H.A. (1965). 'Psychological Differentiation and Forms of Pathology', *J. abn. Psychol.*, *70*, 317-36.

Yakovleva, V.V. (1938). 'Determination of Mobility of the Nervous Processes in the Dog by Means of a Double Transformation of the Conditioned Stimulus', *Trudy Fiziol Labor. I.P. Pavlova, 8.*

Yepes, L., Balka, E., Winsberg, B. and Bialer, I. (1977). 'Amitriptyline and Methylphenidate Treatment of Behaviourally Disordered Children', *J. child Psychol. Psychiat.*, *18*, 9-52.

Yule, W. and Hemsley D. (1977) Single-case method in medical psychology in S. Rachman (ed.), *Contributions to medical psychology*, Pergammon, London.

Zhorov, P.A. and Yermolayeva-Tomina, L.B. (1972) Concerning the relation between extraversion and the strength of the nervous system, in V.D. Nebylitsyn and J.A. Gray (eds), *Biological bases of individual behaviour*, Academic Press, New York.

Index